GERIATRIC EMERGENT/ URGENT AND AMBULATORY CARE

THE POCKET NP

Sheila Sanning Shea, MSN, RN, ANP is an emergency nurse practitioner (ENP) with over 40 years of clinical experience. She works in the Department of Emergency Medicine at St. Mary Medical Center in Long Beach, California. Ms. Shea established an emergency clinical fellowship for nurse practitioners and physician assistants that includes both didactic and clinical experiences. Ms. Shea is widely published and is an author and reviewer for the *Advanced Emergency Nursing Journal*, and was a contributing author to the *Emergency Nurses Core Curriculum* and *Certified Emergency Nurse Review*. Ms. Shea has taught NPs locally and nationally on a variety of emergent and urgent care topics.

Karen Sue Hoyt, PhD, RN, FNP-BC, ENP-C, FAEN, FAANP, FAAN, is an emergency nurse practitioner (ENP) and a professor and director of the NP/ENP programs at the Hahn School of Nursing and Health Science at the University of San Diego. Dr. Hoyt has several peer-reviewed books and publications on clinical practice, research, and management/leadership topics. In 2006, she established the first *Advanced Emergency Nursing Journal*. She conceptualized and has implemented a 2-day course for training ENPs and a train-the-trainer course for NP faculty. She has taught minor procedures workshops for NPs/PAs across the country. As a consultant and educator, she has also written ENP continuing education programs. Dr. Hoyt spearheaded *The Delphi Study on Competencies for NPs in Emergency Care* and serves as an item writer for the American Academy Nurse Practitioners Certification Board. She is the former Chair of the NP Validation Committee for the American Academy of Emergency Nurse Practitioners.

Renee Semonin Holleran, PhD, RN, FNP-BC, CEN, CCRN (Emeritus), CFRN and CTRN (retired), FAEN, has practiced for over 35 years in emergency care. Dr. Holleran is a nurse practitioner at the Integrative Pain Management, Veterans Health Administration in Salt Lake City, Utah. She also practices at the Hope Free Clinic in Midvale, Utah. Dr. Holleran is the former editor of the *Journal of Emergency Nursing* and currently serves on the board of directors of the *Advanced Emergency Nursing Journal*. She is a past recipient of the AJN Book Award in prehospital nursing.

GERIATRIC EMERGENT/ URGENT AND AMBULATORY CARE

THE POCKET NP

SECOND EDITION

Sheila Sanning Shea, MSN, RN, ANP

Karen Sue Hoyt, PhD, RN, FNP-BC, ENP-C, FAEN, FAANP, FAAN

Renee Semonin Holleran, PhD, RN, FNP-BC, CEN, CCRN (Emeritus), CFRN and CTRN (retired), FAEN

SPRINGER PUBLISHING COMPANY

Springer Publishing Company, LLC
11 West 42nd Street, New York, NY 10036
www.springerpub.com
connect.springerpub.com/

Acquisitions Editor: Elizabeth Nieginski
Compositor: Diacritech

ISBN: 978-0-8261-5174-2
ebook ISBN: 978-0-8261-5175-9
DOI: 10.1891/9780826151759

21 22 23 / 5 4 3

The author and the publisher of this Work have made every effort to use sources believed to be reliable to provide information that is accurate and compatible with the standards generally accepted at the time of publication. Because medical science is continually advancing, our knowledge base continues to expand. Therefore, as new information becomes available, changes in procedures become necessary. We recommend that the reader always consult current research and specific institutional policies before performing any clinical procedure or delivering any medication. The author and publisher shall not be liable for any special, consequential, or exemplary damages resulting, in whole or in part, from the readers' use of, or reliance on, the information contained in this book. The publisher has no responsibility for the persistence or accuracy of URLs for external or third-party Internet websites referred to in this publication and does not guarantee that any content on such websites is, or will remain, accurate or appropriate.

Library of Congress Cataloging-in-Publication Data
Library of Congress Control Number: 2020902204

Sheila Sanning Shea: https://orcid.org/0000-0001-9163-7653
Karen Sue Hoyt: https://orcid.org/0000-0003-4810-2308
Renee Semonin Holleran: https://orcid.org/0000-0002-5929-6657

CONTENTS

PREFACE

The *Geriatric Emergent/Urgent and Ambulatory Care: The Pocket NP* is the result of three decades of our experiences as ENPs. We often found our pockets filled with scribbled notes that included tidbits of things—"Don't Miss!" items and important "Tips" and essential information to include in the history and physical documentation. Although we had many excellent medical reference textbooks, we identified the need for a quick reference guide that had an easy-to-use framework for the most commonly encountered problems seen in the emergency, medical screening, fast-track, and/or primary care settings.

The guide focuses on the care of the geriatric patient and is arranged in a logical head-to-toe format that includes the history and physical examination, as well as essential medical decision-making considerations. Templates for "Dictation/Documentation" are provided to assist the clinician with the development of a concise and logical patient record. Also included are frequently used illustrations for anatomical reference.

HOW TO USE THIS GUIDE

Use appropriate sections of the "Geriatric Adult Trauma" or "Geriatric Adult Medical" template defaults to document basic normal findings. Delete any portion of the template that was not examined or is not pertinent to a specific patient. Mix and match portions of various templates to meet your needs and the components of the physical exam.

Fine-tune your assessment skills using the specific dictation/documentation templates for focused patient problems such as "knee pain."

Demonstrate your critical thinking skills by expanding and polishing your "Medical Decision Making."

"Dictation/Documentation Guidelines" are designed as an outline to ensure that all critical elements of the patient record are addressed.

This guide is just that—a guide. It is intended as a quick reference tool only and it is not meant to be a complete review or definitive guide to clinical practice and patient management. The management options are based on current evidence for best practices. However, emergency medicine is an ever-changing specialty and the user of this guide is encouraged to consult other sources to confirm all medication indications, contraindications, side effects, and dosing prior to administration. The authors and publisher specifically disclaim any liability for errors or omissions found here or within, or for any misuse or treatment errors.

Sheila Sanning Shea
Karen Sue Hoyt

ABBREVIATIONS*

AAA	Abdominal aortic aneurysm	CABG	Coronary artery bypass graft
ABC	Airway breathing circulation	CAD	Coronary artery disease
Abd	Abdomen/abdominal	CAM	Confusion assessment method
ABG	Arterial blood gas	CAP	Community acquired pneumonia
ABO	Blood type groups		
Abx	Antibiotics	CAUTI	Catheter associated urinary tract infection
ACC	Assisted care center		
ACE	Angiotensin converting enzyme	CBC	Complete blood count
		CC	Chief complaint
ACI	Aftercare instructions	CFL	Calcaneofibular ligament
ACL	Anterior cruciate ligament	Chem Panel	Chemistry panel
ACS	Acute coronary syndrome	CHF	Congestive heart failure
ADH	Antidiuretic hormone	CKD	Chronic kidney disease
ADL	Activities of daily living	CMS	Circulation/motor/sensation
ADR	Adverse drug reactions	CMT	Cervical motion tenderness
AECB	Acute exacerbation chronic bronchitis	CN	Cranial nerves (I–XII)
		CNS	Central nervous system
AFib	Atrial fibrillation	C/O	Complains of
AGE	Acute gastroenteritis	CO	Carbon monoxide
AIDS	Acquired immunodeficiency syndrome	COPD	Chronic obstructive pulmonary disease
ALOC	Altered level of consciousness	CP	Chest pain
AMI	Acute myocardial infarction	CPAP	Continuous positive airway pressure
AMS	Altered mental status		
A&O	Alert and oriented	CPK-MB	Creatine phosphokinase-MB
AP	Antero posterior	CPPD	Calcium pyrophosphate dihydrate deposition disease
APD	Afferent pupillary defect		
Appy	Appendicitis	CrCl	Creatinine clearance
ASA	Acetylsalicylic acid/aspirin	CRF	Chronic renal failure
Assoc	Associated	CRP	C-reactive protein
ATFL	Anterior talofibular ligament	C&S	Culture and sensitivity
		CSF	Cerebrospinal fluid
AVN	Avascular necrosis	CST	Cavernous sinus thrombosis
AVP	Arteriovenous pressure	CT	Computerized tomography
BID	Twice a day	CTA	Clear to auscultation
BM	Bowel movement	CV	Cardiovascular
BMI	Body mass index	CVA	Cerebral vascular accident
BMP	Basic metabolic panel	CVA/CVAT	Costovertebral angle/costovertebral angle tenderness
BNP	B-type natriuretic peptide		
BO	Bowel obstruction		
B/P	Blood pressure	CVD	Cardiovascular disease
BPH	Benign prostatic hypertrophy	CVP	Central venous pressure
BPPV	Benign paroxysmal positional vertigo	Cx	Culture
		CXR	Chest x-ray
BPV	Benign positional vertigo	D	Day
BS	Bowel sounds	D5LR	Dextrose 5% lactated Ringer's
BSA	Burn surface area	D5NS	Dextrose 5% in 0.9% saline
BUN	Blood urea nitrogen	D10	Dextrose 10%
Ca	Calcium	D&C	Dilation and curettage
CA	Cancer	D/C	Diarrhea/constipation

*The abbreviations used in this book may not be accepted medical abbreviations.

DDD	Degenerative disc disease	GERD	Gastroesophageal reflux disease
DDx	Differential diagnoses	GI	Gastrointestinal
DFA	Direct fluorescent antigen	GSW	Gunshot wound
DI	Diabetes insipidus	gtts	Drops
DIC	Disseminated intravascular coagulopathy	GU	Genitourinary
DIP	Distal interphalangeal	GYN	Gynecologic
DJD	Degenerative joint disease	HA	Headache
DKA	Diabetic ketoacidosis	Hct	Hematocrit
DM	Diabetes mellitus	HCTZ	Hydrochlorothiazide
DMARD	Disease-modifying antirheumatic drug	HEENT	Head/eyes/ears/nose/throat
DNR	Do not resuscitate	Heme	Hematologic
DS	Double strength	Hep	Hepatitis
DSD	Dry sterile dressing	Hgb	Hemoglobin
DTRs	Deep tendon reflexes	HgbA1c	Hemoglobin A1c/ glycohemoglobin (for DM)
DVT	Deep vein thrombosis	HbS	Hemoglobin S
Dx	Diagnosis	HHN	Hand held nebulizer
ED	Emergency department	HHS	Hyperosmolar hyperglycemic state
EDLC	End-of-life care		
EGD	Esophagogastroduodenoscopy	Hib	Haemophilus influenzae type b
EH	Epidural hematoma		
EKG	Electrocardiogram	HIV	Human immunodeficiency virus
ELISA	Enzyme-linked immunosorbent assay		
ENT	Ear, nose, and throat	HM	Hand motion
EOM/EOMI	Extra ocular movements/extra ocular movements intact	HOB	Head of bed
		H&P	History and physical
ESR	Erythrocyte sedimentation rate	HPF	High powered field
		HPI	History of present illness
ETOH	Ethanol (alcohol)	HSM	Hepatosplenomegaly
ETT	Endotracheal tube	HSP	Henoch-Schonlein purpura
Exac	Exacerbation	HSV	Herpes simplex virus
Extrems	Extremities	HTN	Hypertension
FAST	Focused assessment of sonography in trauma	HX	History
		HZV	Herpes zoster virus
FB	Foreign body	IADL	Instrumental activities of daily living
F/C	Fever/chills		
FDP	Flexor digitorum profundus	IBD/IBS	Inflammatory bowel disease/ irritable bowel syndrome
FDS	Flexor digitorum superficialis		
FH	Family history	ICH	Intracranial hemorrhage
FHCS	Fitz-Hugh-Curtis syndrome	ICP	Intracranial pressure
FI	Fecal incontinence	I&D	Incision and drainage
FOOSH	Fall on outstretched hand	IM	Intramuscular
FROM	Full range of motion	Inj	Injury
FBS	Fasting blood sugar	inpt	Inpatient
FTC	Full to confrontation	INR	International normalized ratio
FTI	Free thyroxine index	IO	Inferior oblique
F/U	Follow-up	IOP	Intraocular pressure
FX	Fracture	IP	Interphalangeal
GB	Gallbladder	IR	Inferior rectus
GBS	Group B *Streptococcus*	ITP	Idiopathic thrombocytopenic purpura
GC	Gonococcal/gonorrhea		
GCS	Glasgow Coma Scale		

IV	Intravenous
IVDA	Intravenous drug abuse
IVP	Intravenous push
I	
IVPB	Intravenous piggyback
JLT	Joint line tenderness
JVD	Jugular venous distention
K+	Potassium
KUB	Kidneys, ureters, and bladder
L	Liter
LBBB	Left bundle branch block
LBP	Lower back pain
LCL	Lateral collateral ligament
LFT	Liver function tests
LLQ	Left lower quadrant
LMWH	Low molecular weight heparin
LNMP	Last normal menstrual period
LOC	Loss of consciousness
LP	Lumbar puncture
LR	Lateral rectus
L/R	Left/right
LS	Lumbosacral
LSpine	Lumbosacral spine
LUQ	Left upper quadrant
LVAD	Left ventricular assist device
LVF	Left ventricular failure
LVH	Left ventricular hypertrophy
MAP	Mean arterial pressure
MCL	Medial collateral ligament
MD	Medical doctor
MDM	Medical decision making
Meds	Medications
MI	Myocardial infarction
MME	Mini mental exam
MMM	Mucous membranes moist
MOI	Mechanism of injury
MOLST	Medical orders for life sustaining treatment
MR	Medial rectus
MRA	Magnetic resonance angiography
MRI	Magnetic resonance imaging
MRN	Medical record number
MRSA	Methicillin resistant *Staphylococcus aureus*
MSK	Musculoskeletal
MTBI	Mild traumatic brain injury
MTP	Metatarsophalangeal (joint)
MVC	Motor vehicle crash
NaCl	Sodium chloride
NEXUS	National emergency x-radiology utilization study
NGT	Nasogastric tube
NLP	No light perception
Non Cox	Non Cox inhibitors
NPO	Nothing by mouth
NS	Normal saline
NSAIDs	Nonsteroidal anti-inflammatory drugs
NT	Nontender
NTG	Nitroglycerin
N/V	Nausea/vomiting
N/V/D	Nausea/vomiting/diarrhea
NWB	Nonweight bearing
O_2 Sat	Oxygen saturation/pulse oximetry
OA	Osteoarthritis
OB	Occult blood
OD	Overdose
OLDCART	Onset, location, duration, characteristics, aggravating factors, relieving factors, treatment
Onc	Oncology
ORIF	Open reduction internal fixation
OTC	Over-the-counter
PAD	Peripheral arterial disease
Palp	Palpate/palpitations
PAT	Paroxysmal atrial tachycardia
PCL	Posterior cruciate ligament
PCN	Penicillin
PCP	Primary care physician
PCR	Polymerase chain reaction
PE	Pulmonary embolism
Ped	Pediatrician
PE	Physical exam
PERC	Pulmonary embolism risk factors
PERRLA	Pupils equal and round, reactive to light and accommodation
PID	Pelvic inflammatory disease
PIP	Proximal interphalangeal
PMD	Primary medical doctor
PMH	Past medical history
PMN	Polymorphonuclear
PNA	Pneumonia
PND	Paroxysmal nocturnal dyspnea
PO	Per os (by mouth)
POF	Position of function
POLST	Physician orders for life sustaining treatment
PR	Per the rectum
PRN	As needed
Prob	Problem
ProT	Protime

PSH	Past surgical history/surgical history	STEMI	ST elevation myocardial infarction
Pt/Pts	Patient/Patients	STI	Sexually transmitted infection
PT	Point tenderness	STS	Soft tissue swelling
PTFL	Posterior talofibular ligament	SXS	Symptoms
PTT	Partial thromboplastin time	T3	Triiodothyronine
PTU	Propylthiouracil	T4	Free thyroxine
PUD	Peptic ulcer disease	Ta	Tonometry applanation
PVK	Penicillin V potassium	TAD	Thoracic aortic dissection
PWD	Pink/warm/dry	TB	Tuberculosis
QD	Once per day	TBI	Traumatic brain injury
QID	Four times per day or every six hours	TBSA	Total body surface area
		T&C	Type & crossmatch
RA	Rheumatoid arthritis	tDap	Tetanus diphtheria acellular pertussis
RAI	Radioactive Iodine		
RAIU	Radioactive iodine uptake	TEN	Toxic epidermal necrolysis
Rh	Rhesus factor	TENS	Transcutaneous electrical nerve stimulation
RICE	Rest/ice/compression/elevation		
		TFL	Talofibular ligament
R/L	Right/left	TIA	Transient ischemic attack
RLQ	Right lower quadrant	TID	Three times per day
RMSF	Rocky mountain spotted fever	TM	Tympanic membrane
R/O	Rule/out	TMJ	Temporomandibular joint
ROM	Range of motion	TMP/SMX	Trimethoprim (TMP) sulfamethoxazole (SMX)
ROS	Review of systems		
RPR	Rapid plasma reagin	TOA	Tubo-ovarian abscess
RRR	Regular rate and rhythm	TPO	Thyroid peroxidase
RUQ	Right upper quadrant	T&S	Type & screen
SAH	Subarachnoid hemorrhage	TSH	Thyroid stimulating hormone
SaO2	Oxygen saturation (pulse oximetry)		
		TSI	Thyroid-stimulating immunoglobulin
SBO	Small bowel obstruction		
SBP	Systolic blood pressure	TSS	Toxic shock syndrome
SCD	Sickle cell disease	TTP	Tender to palpation
SDH	Subdural hematoma	TUG	Timed up and go
SH	Social history	TV	Tidal volume
SI	Sacroiliac	UA	Urinalysis
SIADH	Syndrome of inappropriate antidiuretic hormone	UCG	Urine chorionic gonadotropin
		UI	Urinary incontinence
SIRS	Systemic inflammatory response syndrome	Ultz	Ultrasound
		UOP	Urine output
SJS	Stevens-Johnson syndrome	URI	Upper respiratory infection
SLE	Systemic lupus erythematosus/slit lamp exam	UTI	Urinary tract infection
		Utox	Urine toxicology
SLR	Straight leg raise	V/A	Visual/Acuity
SNF	Skilled nursing facility	VBG	Venous blood gas
SNT	Soft nontender	V/D	Vomiting/diarrhea
SO	Superior oblique	VF	Visual fields
SOB	Shortness of breath	VS	Vital signs
SR	Superior rectus	VSS	Vital signs stable
SSKI	Potassium iodide	WBCs	White blood cells
SSRI	Selective serotonin reuptake inhibitor	WDWN	Well-developed, well-nourished
SSS	Scalded skin syndrome	WNL	Within normal limits

DICTATION/DOCUMENTATION GUIDELINES

GENERAL
The pt is alert and oriented, well appearing, appropriately dressed, oriented, in no acute distress

VITAL SIGNS
Note vital signs and interpret as normal or abnormal, pulse oxygen interpretation, weight in kg. Pts older than 65 years may have a B/P of 140/90, which is within normal limits, and pts older than 80 years may have a B/P of 150/90 unless there are other comorbidities such as CKD or diabetes. Alterations in pulse, such as bradycardia, may be the result of medications, especially beta-blockers

SKIN
Warm, dry, pink without rash. Good texture and turgor. No skin breakdown or decubitus ulcer

HEENT
- **Head:** normocephalic
- **Eyes:** sclera and conjunctivae clear. Pinguecula, a yellowish triangular nodule in the bulbar conjunctiva on either side of the iris, may be present on either the nasal or temporal side. Corneal arcus or a thin grayish white arc or circle close to the edge of the cornea. Cataracts may be present. PERRLA. Extraocular movements are intact
- **Ears:** patent canals. Tympanic membranes clear. Tophi may be present on the helix or antihelix of the ear from chronic gout
- **Nose/Face:** without rhinorrhea, face symmetrical; asymmetry may be related to a new or old CVA; decreased facial mobility may be present related to Parkinson's disease
- **Mouth/Throat:** mucous membranes are moist. Tongue symmetrical. Teeth present or absent, upper or lower plates, with or without significant decay. Posterior pharynx clear without erythema, lesions, or exudate

NECK
Supple without any thyromegaly or adenopathy, trachea midline. No bruits or jugular vein distention. No noted dysphagia or drooling

CHEST
No accessory muscle use, normal AP diameter, increased AP diameter (barrel chest), kyphosis, pectus excavatum. Female breasts more flaccid and pendulous. Gynecomastia may be present in the male older pt from hormone or medication influence

HEART
Regular rate and rhythm, no murmurs, gallops, or rubs; peripheral pulses present and equal. If an irregular heart rate is present, may be atrial fibrillation if it is irregularly irregular. An S_4 may be heard in healthy older people, suggestive of decreased ventricular compliance and impaired ventricular filling. A systolic aortic murmur may be heard and is usually related to the thickening of the aortic cusps with fibrous tissue due to aging

ABDOMEN
Protruding, soft, nontender without masses, guarding, and rebound tenderness may be decreased or absent due to aging, blunting these responses. Bowel sounds active or hypoactive. No hepatosplenomegaly

BACK
Without spinal or CVA tenderness

(cont.)

DICTATION/DOCUMENTATION GUIDELINES (cont.)

MUSCULOSKELETAL
Limbs look longer in proportion to the trunk. Decreased tensile strength may be noted because of age or chronic disease such as osteoarthritis

GU
Urinary continence or incontinence. Perineal skin breakdown
Female: pubic hair loss, labia and clitoris decreased in size, vaginal opening short and narrow, vaginal mucosa thin, pale, and dry

PELVIC
Uterus and ovaries diminished in size. Protrusion of bladder or rectum into vaginal vault may be noted
Male: penis decreased in size, testicles noted lower in the scrotum, prostate enlarged, soft to firm

RECTAL
Normal tone. No rectal wall tenderness. Stool is brown and heme negative

EXTREMITIES
Full range of motion may be diminished and crepitus noted. Good to decreased strength bilaterally. Evidence of upper and lower extremity rigidity. No clubbing, cyanosis, or edema. Peripheral pulses intact, dorsalis pedal pulse may not be palpated, posterior tibial pulse present. Presence of vascular changes, varicose veins, vascular ulcers, pigmented skin, hair loss. Peripheral edema-pitting or nonpitting, anterior tibia or feet. Sensation intact or decreased. Rheumatoid arthritis, Bouchard's nodes noted in PIP area, in osteoarthritis Heberden's nodes common in DIP joints. Tophi may be present in toes and finger joints related to gout. Swan neck deformities of the joint are related to rheumatoid arthritis

NEURO
Pt is alert, oriented or disoriented, dressed appropriately or signs of poor hygiene, such as lack of bathing, dirty hair and nails, clothes not clean, engaging in no acute distress. Speech clear. Brief MME if indicated, that is, "What is the year, date, or month? Where are you—hospital or department?" Three word recall.

- Cranial nerve II to XII intact
- Motor sensory exam nonfocal
- Tremor—at rest or intentional
- Moves all extremities
- **Gait:** pt is or is not able to get up from a sitting position with or without assistance. Steady, unsteady, use of an assistance device to ambulate
- **Romberg**
- **Balance:** Normal or abnormal

GENERAL
The pt is well appearing for age. Alert and oriented and conversant in no apparent distress

VITAL SIGNS
Note vital signs and interpret as normal or abnormal, pulse ox interpretation, weight in kg. *Pts older than 65 may have a B/P of 140/90, which is within normal limits, and pts older than 80 years may have B/P of 150/90.* Alterations in pulse, such as bradycardia, may be the result of medications, especially beta-blockers. Note whether pacemaker or internal defibrillator present

MEDICAL TEMPLATE

GENERAL
The pt is alert and oriented, well appearing, appropriately dressed, oriented in no acute distress or dressed inappropriately or signs of poor hygiene (e.g., lack of bathing, dirty hair/nails, clothes)

VITAL SIGNS
Note vital signs and interpret as normal or abnormal, pulse ox interpretation, weight in kg. Pts older than 65 may have a B/P at 140/90, which is within normal limits, and pts older than 80 years may have a B/P at 150/90. Alterations in pulse, such as bradycardia, may be the result of medications, especially beta-blockers

SKIN
Warm, dry, pink without rash. Good texture and turgor

HEENT
- **Head:** normocephalic
- **Eyes:** sclera and conjunctivae clear. Pinguecula, a yellowish triangular nodule in bulbar conjunctiva. Corneal arcus/thin grayish-white arc/circle (edge of cornea). Cataracts. PERRLA. EOMIs
- **Ears:** patent canals. Tympanic membranes clear. Tophi may be present on the helix or antihelix of the ear from chronic gout
- **Nose/Face:** without rhinorrhea, face symmetrical, asymmetry may be related to a new or old CVA, decreased facial mobility may be present related to Parkinson's disease
- **Mouth/Throat:** mucous membranes are moist. Tongue symmetrical. Teeth present or absent, upper or lower plates, with or without significant decay. Posterior pharynx clear without erythema, lesions, or exudate

NECK
Supple without any thyromegaly or adenopathy, trachea midline. No bruits or jugular vein distention. No noted dysphagia or drooling

CHEST
No accessory muscle use, normal AP diameter, increased AP diameter (barrel chest), kyphosis, pectus excavatum
Females: breasts: flaccid, pendulous
Males: gynecomastia

HEART
Regular rate and rhythm, no murmurs, gallops, or rubs; peripheral pulses present and equal. AFib: irregularly irregular. S_4: decreased ventricular compliance and impaired ventricular filling. Systolic aortic murmur: thickening of aortic cusps with fibrous tissue caused by aging

ABDOMEN
Protruding, soft, NT without masses, guarding and rebound tenderness may be decreased or absent in the abd as a result of aging, blunting these responses. Bowel sounds active or hypoactive. No hepatosplenomegaly

BACK
Without spinal or CVA tenderness

(cont.)

MEDICAL TEMPLATE (cont.)

MUSCULOSKELETAL
Limbs look longer in proportion to the trunk. Decreased tensile strength may be noted as a result of age or chronic disease such as osteoarthritis

GU
Urinary continence or incontinence noted
   Female: pubic hair loss, labia and clitoris decreased in size, vaginal opening short and narrow, vaginal mucosa-thin pale and dry

PELVIC
Uterus and ovaries diminished in size. Protrusion of bladder or rectum into vaginal vault may be noted
   Male: penis decreased in size, testicles noted lower in the scrotum, prostate enlarged, soft to firm

RECTAL
Normal tone. No rectal wall tenderness. Stool is brown and heme negative

EXTREMITIES
Full range of motion may be diminished and crepitus noted. Good to decreased strength bilaterally. Evidence of upper and lower extremity rigidity. No clubbing, cyanosis, or edema. Peripheral pulses intact, dorsalis pedal pulse may not be palpated, posterior tibial pulse present. Presence of vascular changes, varicose veins, vascular ulcers, pigmented skin, hair loss. Peripheral edema-pitting or nonpitting, anterior tibia or feet. Sensation intact or decreased. Rheumatoid arthritis, Bouchard's nodes noted in PIP area, in osteoarthritis Heberden's nodes common in DIP joints. Tophi may be present in toes and finger joints related to gout

NEURO
- MME as indicated
- Pt is alert, oriented or disoriented. Speech clear
- CN II to XII intact
- Motor sensory exam nonfocal
- Tremor—at rest or intentional
- Moves all extremities
- Gait: pt is or is not able to get up from a sitting position with or without assistance. Steady, unsteady, use of assistance device to ambulate
- Romberg
- Balance: normal or abnormal

TRAUMA TEMPLATE

GENERAL
The pt is well-appearing for age. Alert and oriented and conversant in no apparent distress

VITAL SIGNS
Note vital signs and interpret as normal or abnormal, pulse ox interpretation, weight in kg. Pts older than 65 may have a B/P at 140/90, which is within normal limits, and pts older than 80 years may have B/P at 150/90. Alterations in pulse, such as bradycardia, may be the result of medications, especially beta-blockers. Note whether pacemaker or internal defibrillator is present

SKIN
Warm, dry, no obvious injuries

HEENT
- **Head:** normocephalic, atraumatic without palpable deformities
- **Eyes:** pupils equal, round, and reactive to light. Note whether cataracts may be present No periorbital ecchymosis or step-off. Extraocular movements are intact
- **Ears:** patent canals. Tympanic membranes clear. No Battle's sign. No hemotympanum
- **Nose/Face:** atraumatic. There is no septal hematoma. Facial bones nontender to palpation and stable with attempts at manipulation
- **Mouth/Throat:** no intraoral trauma. Teeth, if present, and mandible are intact

NECK
No midline point tenderness, step-off, or deformity to firm palpation of posterior cervical spine. Trachea midline. Carotids equal. No masses. No JVD. Full range of motion of neck without limitation or pain

CHEST
No surface trauma. Nontender without crepitus or deformity. No palpable subcutaneous air. Lungs have good tidal volume for stated age with normal breath sounds

HEART
Regular rate and rhythm or rhythm noted as normal for the pt. Tones are normal and clear

ABDOMEN
No abrasions or ecchymosis or surface trauma. No distention. Nontender to palpation, no guarding, rebound tenderness, or rigidity. No masses. Bowel sounds are active

BACK
No contusions, ecchymosis, or surface trauma. No distention. Nontender to palpation without step-off or deformity to firm midline palpation. No CVAT or flank ecchymosis

GU
Normal external genitalia with no blood at the meatus. No swelling or tenderness

PELVIS
Nontender to palpation and stable to compression. Femoral pulses strong and equal

RECTAL
Normal tone. No rectal wall tenderness. Stool is brown and heme negative

(cont.)

TRAUMA TEMPLATE (cont.)

EXTREMITIES

No surface trauma. Full range of motion without limitation or pain. Good strength in all extremities for stated age. Sensations to light touch intact. All peripheral pulses are intact and equal based on pt's physical condition. No evidence of hip shortening or external rotation

NEURO

A&O × 4. GCS 15, 4/6/5. CN II–XII intact. Motor sensory exam nonfocal. Reflexes are symmetric

REVIEW OF SYSTEMS

The ROS is not the same as the HPI, which addresses pertinent positives and negatives of the chief complaint. The ROS is an "inventory" of organ systems used to investigate the pt's general state of health

GENERAL
F/C, myalgias, fatigue/lethargy/malaise, sweats, weight loss/gain, recent fall, ability to walk and move, hygiene and mood

ACTIVITIES OF DAILY LIVING
Bathing, dressing, toileting, transferring, continence, feeding, managing money, use of communication devices, shopping, preparing food, housekeeping, laundry, transportation (able to drive); managing medications

DERM
Rash, lesions, itching, carcinoma

NEURO
HA, dizziness, vertigo, weakness, trouble with speech or balance, seizures, repetitive behaviors, confusion

EYE
Blurred/double vision, eye pain, flashing lights, pain, drainage, cataracts, glasses/contacts, trouble with glare or dim light, night vision

ENT/NECK
Earache, ringing in ears, decreased hearing/hearing aid, nasal congestion, nosebleeds, sore throat, hoarseness, difficulty swallowing or drooling, dry mouth, dental problems, dentures, taste, neck pain, stiffness, swollen glands

RESP
SOB, wheezing, pleuritic chest pain, cough/sputum, hemoptysis, orthopnea, paroxysmal nocturnal dyspnea

CV
Chest pain, palpitations/irregular heartbeat, lightheaded/dizzy, syncope, diaphoresis, exertional dyspnea, paroxysmal nocturnal dyspnea, leg pain/swelling

GI
Abd pain, N/V, D/C, loss of appetite, heartburn, hematemesis, melena, jaundice, bowel changes

GU/GYN
Dysuria, frequency, urgency, hematuria, flank pain, testicular pain/swelling, penile discharge, vaginal bleeding or discharge, sexual activity

MSK
Joint pain/swelling/stiffness, leg pain or swelling, back pain

HEME
Bruising or bleeding, petechiae, anemia, clots, transfusions

ENDOCRINE
Polyuria, polydipsia, cold/heat intolerance

PSYCH
Hallucinations, depression, suicidal/homicidal ideation, dementia

ALLERGIC/IMMUNIZATIONS
No allergies/immunizations

FALL ASSESSMENT

HX
- Falls (single fall within the last 12 months should be evaluated)
- LOC
- Time spent down before rescue
- Melena
- Current meds
- Use of assistive device
- Current footwear
- Visual problems
- Neurological disease (e.g., Parkinson's disease)
- Cardiac disease
- Postural hypotension
- Environmental hazards
- Inc in urinary frequency or urgency

PMH
- History of substance abuse, ETOH
- Diminished vision and/or hearing
- DJD
- Frequent UTI
- Constipation

PE
- **General:** alert, disoriented, confused, tremulous, arousable, agitated, lethargic, stuporous, delirious, comatose. Recognition/interaction with family members or significant others. Hygiene; trauma; odors (ETOH, acetone, almonds)
- **VS and SaO$_2$:** fever/hypothermia, brady/tachycardia, resp depression, hypo/hyperventilation
- **Skin:** texture, turgor, rash, petechiae/purpura, jaundice, needle marks
- **HEENT:**
  - **Head:** surface trauma
  - **Eyes:** PERRLA, fixed/dilated, icterus, EOMI, ptosis, fundi (papilledema, retinal hemorrhage)
  - **Ears:** canals patent, hemotympanum, CSF leak
  - **Nose:** CSF leak
  - **Face:** symmetric, weakness
  - **Mouth/Throat:** gag reflex, tongue symmetry
- **Neck:** meningismus, nuchal rigidity, thyroid
- **Chest:** CTA, heart RRR, resp effort
- **Abd:** soft, NT, pulsatile mass, ascites, hepatomegaly, suprapubic TTP, or distension
- **Extrems:** FROM, NT, strength and sensation, weakness, tremors, asterixis (liver hand flap), rigidity
- **Rectal:** tone, occult blood, melena
- **Neuro:** A&O × 4, GCS 15- 4/6/5, CN II–XII, focal neuro deficit, DTRs, pathological reflexes, speech/gait, Romberg, pronator drift, speech clear, gait steady, spontaneous or uncontrolled movements, abnormal posturing, flaccid. Gait impairment: joint stiffness, numbness, spasticity, shuffling steps, reduced arm swinging, ataxia, freezing of gait. Timed Up and Go (TUG)—rising from the chair, walking 3 m, turning, and returning to sit in the chair. Recommended this should be accomplished in >14 seconds

(cont.)

FALL ASSESSMENT (cont.)

MDM/DDX
MDM includes ruling out trauma, such as **head or cervical spine injury;** evaluate for **hip and/or pelvic fractures,** evaluate for other causes, such as **neurologic** and/or **cardiac disease** (e.g., arrhythmias), orthostatic hypotension, UTI, constipation, or problems with medication usage

MANAGEMENT
- Identification of significant injuries
- CT head/spine
- Pelvic/hip x-rays as indicated
- EKG
- CBC, chemistries
- UA, Cx
- Medication levels when indicated
- Admit as indicated
- Consults as needed
- TUG should be assessed before discharge—rising from the chair, walking 3 m, turning, and returning to sit in the chair. Admission may need to be considered if pt is not in a safe environment
- Fall prevention
- Education, including environmental risks, appropriate footwear, when to take medications that may cause dizziness, and importance of getting up slowly when postural hypotension has been identified. Referral for home health care from the ED may be useful if risks are identified.

DICTATION/DOCUMENTATION
- **General:** alert and oriented, confused, nonresponsive. No odors. VSS, no fever or tachycardia
- **VS and SaO$_2$**
- **Skin:** PWD, no lesions or rash, no surface trauma noted
- **HEENT:**
  - **Head:** scalp atraumatic, NT
  - **Eyes:** sclera and conjunctiva clear, corneas grossly clear, PERRLA, EOMI, no nystagmus or disconjugate gaze, no ptosis. Corneal reflex intact. Fundoscopic exam.
  - **Ears:** canals and TMs normal. No hemotympanum or Battle's sign
  - **Nose/Face:** atraumatic, NT, no asymmetry
  - **Mouth/Throat:** MMM, posterior pharynx clear, normal gag reflex, no intraoral trauma
- **Neck:** supple, FROM, NT, no lymphadenopathy, no meningismus
- **Chest:** CTA, no wheezes, rhonchi, rales. Normal TV, no retractions or accessory muscle use. No respiratory depression
- **Heart:** RRR, no murmurs, rubs, or gallops
- **Abd:** soft, NT, pulsatile mass, ascites, hepatosplenomegaly, suprapubic TTP or distension, pelvis stable or unstable
- **Back:** without spinal or CVA tenderness
- **Extrems:** moves all extremities with good strength, distal motor neurovascular intact. Area of injury—see specific injury descriptions
- **Neuro:** A&O × 4, GCS 15, 4/6/5. CN II–XII grossly intact. No focal neurological deficits. Normal muscle strength and tone. Normal DTRs, negative Babinski, normal

(cont.)

FALL ASSESSMENT (cont.)

finger-to-nose coordination or heel-to-shin glide. Speech, gait, Romberg neg, no pronator drift

TIPS

- **Hyponatremia:** older pts are at greater risk for hyponatremia related to medications, renal function, and heart failure. This can cause falls
- **Anticoagulants:** older pts who are on anticoagulants are at risk for bleeding, especially intracerebral hemorrhage. In some institutions, these pts are considered trauma pts and a trauma response may need to be initiated
- **Aging:** dizziness is a common problem with aging and can cause falls. Many times pts have had extensive workups for this with no specific reason found. Pt may need affirmation and referral for evaluation and treatment of this chronic condition

GERIATRIC DEPRESSION SCALE

		Yes	No	SCORE
1.	Are you basically satisfied with life?	0	1	
2.	Have you dropped many activities and interests?	1	0	
3.	Do you feel your life is empty?	1	0	
4.	Do you often get bored?	1	0	1
5.	Are you in good spirits most of the time?		0	0
6.	Are you afraid that something bad is going to happen to you?		1	
7.	Do you feel happy most of the time?	0	1	
8.	Do you often feel helpless?	1	0	
9.	Do you prefer to stay at home rather than going out and doing new things?	1	0	0
10.	Do you feel you have more problems with your memory than most?		1	
11.	Do you think it is wonderful to be alive now?	0	1	
12.	Do you feel pretty worthless the way you are now?	1	0	
13.	Do you feel full of energy?	0	1	0
14.	Do you feel that your situation is hopeless?		1	
15.	Do you think that most people are better off than you are?	1	0	

Score > 5 indicates depression

Source: Geriatric Depression Scale (short form). (n.d.). Retrieved from https://geriatrictoolkit.missouri.edu/cog/GDS_SHORT_FORM.PDF

MEDICATIONS TO BE AVOIDED

Medication	Potential Side Effects
Anticholinergics Over-the-counter cold medications Sleep aids; e.g., doxylamine (Unisom Sleep) Diphenhydramine Hydroxyzine Promethazine	Clearance reduced with advanced age Greater risk of confusion, dry mouth, constipation **Use of diphenhydramine in special situations, such as acute treatment of severe allergic reaction, may be appropriate**
Antispasmodics Dicyclomine (Bentyl) Hyoscyamine Scopolamine	**Note:** May be used in palliative care to decrease excessive secretions
Anti-infective Nitrofurantoin	Potential for pulmonary toxicity, lack of efficacy in pts with Creatinine clearance (CrCl) <60 mL/min due to inadequate urinary concentration of the drug
Cardiovascular Alpha-blockers Prazosin (Minipress) Terazosin	Risk of orthostatic hypotension
Alpha agonists, central Clonidine	May cause orthostatic hypotension, bradycardia, and CNS effects
Antiarrhythmic drugs Amiodarone Flecainide Quinidine Sotalol	Multiple toxicities, including QT prolongation
Dronedarone (Multaq)	May induce congestive heart failure
Digoxin	In heart failure and renal clearance issues may cause toxicity and worsen heart failure
Central nervous system Benzodiazepines	Increased sensitivity to these drugs and slower metabolism of long-acting agents Increased risk of cognitive impairment, delirium, falls, and MVC **May be appropriate for use of seizures, sleep disorders, ethanol withdrawal, procedural anesthesia, end-of-life care**
Gastrointestinal Metoclopramide (Reglan)	Can cause extrapyramidal effects such as tardive dyskinesia

(cont.)

MEDICATIONS TO BE AVOIDED

MEDICATIONS TO BE AVOIDED (cont.)

Medication	Potential Side Effects
Pain Non-COX selective NSAIDs Indomethacin Ketorolac (including parental)	Increased risk of GI bleeding and peptic ulcer disease, especially in pts over the age of 75 Increased risk of bleeding in pts taking steroids, anticoagulants, or antiplatelets

Antipsychotics
First generation:
    Chlorpromazine
    Haloperidol
Second generation:
    Olanzapine
    Quetiapine
    Risperidone
	Increased risk of CVA and increased risk of mortality in pts with major cognitive disorders (dementia)

Skeletal muscle relaxants Carisoprodol (Soma) Cyclobenzaprine (Flexeril) Metaxalone (Skelaxin) Methocarbamol (Robaxin)	Most muscle relaxants are poorly tolerated by older adults because of anticholinergic adverse effects, sedation, unsure of amount of dosage that should be used

Adapted from **American Geriatrics Society:** Beers Criteria Update Expert Panel. (2012). American Geriatrics Society updated Beers Criteria for potentially inappropriate medication use in older adults. *Journal of the American Geriatrics Society.* doi:10.111/j.1532-5415.2012.0323.x

BILLING CONSIDERATIONS

Level 1 Problem Focused	Level 2–3 Expanded Problem Focused	Level 4 or 5 Detailed or Comprehensive
Chief complaint	Chief complaint	Chief complaint
HPI: focused 1–3 elements	HPI: 1–3 elements	HPI: >4 elements OR status of 3 or more chronic or inactive conditions
PMH: none required	PMH	PMH
FH/SH: none required	FH/SH: none required, include if pertinent	FH/SH: detailed
ROS: none required	ROS: 1 element	ROS: 2–10 elements
Exam: focused exam of one body area or organ system	Exam: focused exam of one body area or organ system plus related organ system or symptom	Exam: detailed and comprehensive
MDM: Minimal number of diagnostic or treatment options Minimal or no data reviewed Minimal risk complications, morbidity, or mortality	MDM: Limited number of diagnostic or treatment options Limited or no data reviewed Limited risk complications, morbidity or mortality. (Difference in level 2 or 3 depends on complexity of decision making such as consideration of differential diagnoses)	MDM: Highly complex and detailed

NOTE: Documentation guidelines vary depending on each billing situation. Claims submitted to Medicaid and/or Medicare must adhere to the CMS (Centers for Medicare & Medicaid Services "Documentation Guidelines for Evaluation and Management Services"). Some providers use these guidelines for all payers while others follow the American Medical Association (AMA). Current Procedural Terminology (CPT) and Evaluation and Management (E/M) codes are for nongovernmental payers. Levels of care range from 1 to 5 and in order to "score" a chart for billing a certain level of care and varying numbers of organ systems must be reviewed.

SKIN RASHES/LESIONS

HX

- OLDCART: Onset, Location (distribution and progression), Duration, Characteristics (e.g., pruritic, burning), Aggravating or Relieving factors, and Treatments employed prior to arrival
- F/C, N/V, mucous membrane involvement, palmar/sole involvement
- Swelling of face, eyes, intraoral, trouble swallowing or breathing, wheezing, cough, coryza.
- History of similar episodes
- Possible exposure, potential allergens, travel, risk for MRSA
- Change in medication or medication combination
- Family/friends with similar symptoms, communal living (e.g., care center)
- Drugs esp. meth use, psych HX
- HX of cancer, renal or liver disease, chronic stasis dermatitis
- Zoster vaccination

PE

- **General:** alert, not toxic appearing
- **VS and SaO$_2$:** note if febrile or tachycardic
- **Skin:** PWD
- Note lesion size, shape, color, texture, location, blanching
- **Type:** macular, papular, plaque, wheal, vesicle, pustule, bullae, cyst, nodule, ulcer, fissure, scale
- **Pattern/Distribution:** localized, diffuse, discrete, linear, confluent, annular, grouped, confluent, dermatomal, guttate, zosteriform, reticular, herpetiform, serpiginous, pedun/umbil, multiform, morbilliform, scarlatiniform, reticular crusts, exudates, excoriation
- Edema, erythema, induration, or fluctuance
- Nikolsky sign—outer epidermis easily rubbed off; underlying layer of skin
- **HEENT:**
  - **Head:** normocephalic, atraumatic, kerion, hair loss
  - **Eyes:** PERRLA, EOMI, sclera and conjunctiva clear, periorbital lesions, STS or erythema
  - **Ears:** canals and TMs normal, pre- or postauricular lymphadenopathy, lesions
  - **Nose:** normal, rhinorrhea. Vesicle at tip of nose (Hutchinson sign) concern for ophthalmic HZV
  - **Face:** symmetric, lesions
  - **Mouth/Throat:** MMM, posterior pharynx clear, mucosal lesions, strawberry tongue, palatine petechiae, vesicles, Koplik spots
- **Neck:** supple, FROM, lymphadenopathy or meningismus
- **Chest:** RRR, no murmur, run, or gallop
- **Abd:** soft, BSA, NT, HSM
- **Back:** spinal or CVAT
- **Extremities:** FROM with good strength, evidence of venous stasis

(cont.)

SKIN RASHES/LESIONS (cont.)

MDM/DDx

Evaluation of dermatologic disorders in the older adult is directed toward identification of potential life-threatening conditions and assessment of contributing factors and possible systemic disease. Senescent changes in aging skin leads to thin, fragile skin that is easily torn and causes delayed healing. Other aging changes include wrinkling, loss of subcutaneous support, hair loss, and thinning. *Pruritus due to dry skin* (**xerosis**) is a very common complaint in the older adult; repeated scratching can lead to excoriation and secondary infection. *Pruritus without rash should prompt investigation of systemic illness* such as **lymphoma, thyroid, renal,** or **liver disease**. *Dry, cracked, fissured skin on the legs* with scales and plaques may be asteatotic **eczema** and is triggered by dehydration or malnutrition; contact dermatitis from soaps or detergents; discontinued corticosteroid therapy; and neurologic disorders. *If generalized,* may indicate underlying **malignancy**.

Impaired venous return in the legs leads to skin changes caused by venous insufficiency and marked by macerated, crusted, and scaly patches, as well as areas of hyperpigmentation, ulceration, and swelling: The result is often a poorly healing wound and increased morbidity in the older adult. *Chronic ulcers* should be evaluated for **squamous cell carcinoma**.

- **Bullous pemphigoid** is a common chronic autoimmune disease in the older adult. Lesions are mildly pruritic and can be nonspecific and dry or erythematous urticarial plaques. Over days to weeks, large tense clear or hemorrhagic subepidermal blisters (bullae) form on extremities; bullae may also form on intact skin areas. The bullae become eroded, crusted, and excoriated with possible purulent drainage. While usually benign, bullous pemphigoid may be associated with malignancy or precipitated by medications, such as ibuprofen, furosemide, enalapril, or drugs containing phenacetin
- **Herpes zoster (shingles)**, caused by the varicella zoster virus, is a common problem in the older adult because of diminished immunity. This unilateral rash results in groups or bands of painful, erythematous vesicles and papules limited to a specific dermatome. It is essential to identify involvement of the ophthalmic branch of the trigeminal nerve, which can affect the cornea and cause blindness; a lesion on the tip of the nose (Hutchinson sign) is a diagnostic clue. Long-term postherpetic neuralgia can be problematic
- Older people have many *precancerous skin lesions*, such as **actinic keratosis, basal or squamous cell carcinomas, and, more rarely, malignant melanoma. Basal cell carcinoma** appears as a superficial, erythematous macule or papule surrounded by telangiectasia or a waxy translucent papule with overlying telangiectasia and central ulceration
- **Squamous cell carcinoma** is usually a tender, erythematous papule, plaque, or nodule with a keratotic scale most often found on sun-exposed areas
- **Melanomas** are atypical pigmented lesions, nodules, or papules, irregularly shaped, tan, or brown that are found all over the body. Areas of sun-damaged skin are at increased risk. Dark brown or black patches found on the palms, soles, or nail beds with a pigmented streak of the cuticle is known as a Hutchinson sign and incidence is highest in adults >65 years of age

(cont.)

SKIN RASHES/LESIONS (cont.)

MANAGEMENT

- OTC topical ointments/creams can be used for minor skin infections (e.g., Bacitracin, Neosporin). When early MRSA is suspected, mupirocin (Bactroban 0.2%) applied BID to the affected area is recommended for 7 to 10 days. For more serious infections, oral, IM, or IV Abx will be used. Treatment with antibiotics will depend on the microorganism (e.g., antibacterials—Clindamycin or Bactrim or Keflex for strep coverage). (Refer to Antibiogram/Antibiotic policy at facility.)
- **Pruritus:** identify cause; topical medications such as low-dose corticosteroids; hydration, avoid prolonged cold or dry conditions. Use moisturizing lotions, such as Aquaphor or Dermisil. If systemic medications used for pruritus, be aware of increased fall risk. Oral steroids may be required in severe cases with dermatology referral
- **Venous insufficiency:** elevation of extremity with compression socks. Consider an ankle–brachial index before ordering compression socks to rule out peripheral arterial disease as a cause of ulcerated area. Overlying dermatitis can be treated with topical steroids and oral antibiotics if infected
- **Bullous pemphigoid:** topical steroids can be used for localized lesions but may need systemic steroids, which need to be used cautiously in older adults to avoid hyperglycemia, HTN, and negative effect on bone density. Specialist consultation may order an immunosuppressive agent such as methotrexate
- **Herpes zoster:** for pts who present within 72 hours of onset of rash, systemic antiviral medication may be indicated and help reduce duration, acute pain, and postherpetic neuralgia
  - Acyclovir is considered a secondary option now. Valacyclovir or famciclovir are recommended as primary. Acyclovir 800 mg i PO 5× per day × 10 days or use valacyclovir or famciclovir
  - **Postherpetic** neuralgia may respond to topical agents such as lidocaine or capsaicin. Other options include opioids, tricyclic antidepressants, and gabapentin. Older adults should receive herpes zoster vaccine, which can help reduce the incidence of the disease and degree of postherpetic neuralgia pain
- **Erythematous:** serious erythematous rashes that cause fever include **TSS** (mucous membranes) and **TEN** (adults). Also consider "Red Man Syndrome," a hypersensitivity reaction to vancomycin. **Maculopapular:** presence of fever may indicate **viral exanthem, drug reaction,** or **pityriasis** (herald patch). In ill-appearing pts with target lesions consider **SJS** or **erythema multiforme**
  - Febrile and ill pts with peripheral erythematous lesions should prompt consideration of **RMSF, syphilis,** or **Lyme disease**
  - More common and benign etiologies are **scabies, eczema, psoriasis, tinea**
- **Vesicular/Bullous:** Diffuse distribution of vesicles or bullae with fever may indicate **varicella, disseminated GC, smallpox,** or **DIC.** Localized lesions point to serious **necrotizing fasciitis** or benign viral etiologies (hand–foot–mouth Dx). Afebrile etiology rashes include **bullous pemphigoid, pemphigus vulgaris, contact dermatitis, HSV, burn injury, dyshidrotic eczema, actinic keratosis: superficial, flat papules may be covered with dry skin**
- **Petechiae or purpura:** palpable petechiae or purpura in ill-appearing pts are very serious findings. Consider **meningococcemia, disseminated GC, endocarditis, RMSF,** or **HSP.** Autoimmune disorders may cause similar lesions but the pt usually appears well. Flat, impalpable lesions may indicate **DIC, TTP, ITP.** Vasculitis, inflammation of the blood vessels, can be caused by a wide variety of disorders

(cont.)

SKIN RASHES/LESIONS (cont.)

PRIMARY LESIONS

- **Macule:** <1 cm (over 1 cm is patch)
- **Papule:** solid raised lesion with distinct borders, <1 cm; may be domed, flat-topped, umbilicated
- **Nodule:** raised solid lesion more than 1 cm (mass >1 cm)
- **Plaque:** solid, raised, flat-topped (plateau) lesion >1 cm in diameter
- **Vesicle:** raised lesions <1 cm in diameter that are filled with clear fluid
- **Pustule:** circumscribed elevated pustular lesions commonly infected
- **Bullae:** circumscribed fluid-filled lesions that are >1 cm in diameter
- **Wheal:** area of edema in the upper epidermis
- **Burrow:** linear lesions produced by infestation of the skin and formation of tunnels

DICTATION/DOCUMENTATION

- **VS and mental status**
- **Skin:** color, temperature, moisture, texture, turgor. Note mucous membrane involvement, blisters, peeling, extensive erythema, presence or absence of purpura/petechiae, or secondary infection. Describe rash or lesions, including location, distribution, and configuration

SEVERE ALLERGIC REACTION/ANAPHYLAXIS

- **General approach and principles of treatment are the same in older and young pts**
- Implications for management are based on age-related side effects, harmful drug interactions, polypharmacy, and cognitive impairment or frailty
- Comorbidities in older adults increase morbidity and mortality related to severe allergic reactions. Potential for drug interactions increases with age and number of meds prescribed. Consider angiotensin-converting enzyme inhibitor angioedema (AC-ACE), which is common if taking ACE meds
- Incidence of adverse drug reactions (ADR) is increased in frail older adults and OD is a concern. Watch for penicillins, cephalosporins, NSAIDs, quinolones, sulfa, nitrofurantoin, heparin, anticonvulsants, chemotherapy
- β-blockers can cause refractory anaphylaxis that is difficult to treat (glucagon may help)
- Use first-generation antihistamines with extreme caution in older adults: increase confusion, sedation, cognitive impairment, and risk of urinary retention. Second-generation antihistamines are metabolized by liver or kidney and may need reduced dosing
- Corticosteroid use can increase the risk of developing DM or ulcers

◯ TIPS

- Medication-related rashes Abx: penicillin, cephalosporins, sulfonamides, vancomycin, nitrofurantoin
- ASA/NSAIDs—use with caution in older adults and lower the dose
- Barbiturates; contrast dyes
- Pain meds with codeine
- Seizure meds: carbamazepine or valproate. Complementary and alternative medications: echinacea
- GREAT MIMICKER: syphilis—early SXS similar to many other rashes

(cont.)

SKIN RASHES/LESIONS (cont.)

DON'T MISS!

Ill pts with:
- hypotension
- meningococcemia
- TSS
- TEN
- SJS
- DIC
- RMSF
- petechiae
- purpura

BURNS

HX

- MOI
- Type of burn, length of exposure to the burn agent, falls, explosions, exposure to chemicals or electrical current
- Time of burn injury
- Possibility of inhalation injury (closed space exposure, carbon monoxide, cyanide)
- Concomitant trauma
- Past medical history
- Tetanus immunization status
- Allergies
- Risk for neglect or inability to care for self

PE

- **General:** level of pain and distress
- **VS and SaO$_2$**
- **Skin:** color, temperature, TBSA, circumferential burns (see "Tips"), depth of burn
- **Superficial (first degree):** epidermis only, red and painful, blanches with pressure
- **Superficial partial thickness (second degree):** epidermis and superficial dermis, painful, red, weeping, blistered, blanches with pressure. May be a **deep partial thickness** (second degree) that is less painful, blisters, patchy red and white, wet to waxy dry, nonblanching
- **Full thickness (third degree):** through epidermis and dermis, lack of sensation, waxy white to leathery grey to charred and black, dry and inelastic, nonblanching
- **HEENT:**
  - **Head:** atraumatic
  - **Eyes:** PERRLA, periorbital STS, erythema, singed lashes, scleral injection, corneal epithelial defect with fluorescein stain under Wood's lamp
  - **Ears:** TMs and canals normal, no STS or erythema
  - **Nose/Face:** singed nasal hairs, facial burns
  - **Mouth/Throat:** burned or swollen lips, drooling, stridor, dysphagia, odor of soot on breath, carbonaceous secretions, intraoral burns
- **Neck:** STS
- **Chest:** tachypnea, dyspnea, retractions, grunting, coughing, wheezing, rhonchi; surface burns
- **Heart:** RRR
- **Abd:** surface trauma, soft, BSA, nontender without guarding or rebound
- **Back:** no spinal or CVAT
- **Pelvis:** nontender to palpation; no erythema, STS, or burn of external genitalia
- **Extremities:** atraumatic, normal strength and tone, no STS, normal peripheral pulses in each limb
- **Neuro:** awake, alert, age-appropriate behavior

(cont.)

BURNS (cont.)

MDM/DDx

Inhalation and airway injuries are priority assessment and management challenges in older patients with burns. Evidence of airway compromise and respiratory distress must be aggressively managed, often requiring early intubation. High-risk symptoms that may indicate the need for intubation include persistent cough, wheezing, or stridor; carbonaceous sputum or severe blistering in the oropharynx; severe facial burns; circumferential neck burns; altered mental status; respiratory distress; and worsening hypoxia or hypercapnia. Older burn pts often have comorbidities that increase the risk of complications and are susceptible to shock due to hypovolemia. Burns to critical areas, such as the face, hands, feet, genitalia, and across major joints, often require transfer to a burn center.

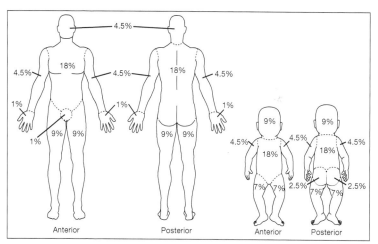

Rule of nines burn chart (adult and child)
Source: Reproduced from Veenema, T. G. (2019). *Disaster nursing and emergency preparedness: For chemical, biological, and radiological terrorism and other hazards* (4th ed.). New York, NY: Springer Publishing Company.

(cont.)

BURNS (cont.)

MANAGEMENT

Major Burns

- Immediate stabilization, ABCs, continuous pulse oximetry, O_2 administration, IV access
- **Fluid administration:** for burns that exceed 15% TBSA use the Parkland formula (4 × weight [kg] × % TBSA burn), administering lactated Ringer's solution. Administer 50% fluid over the first 8 hours, and infuse the remaining fluid over the next 16 hours. Maintenance fluid must also be given concomitantly. Goal is to maintain urine output of 1 mL/kg per hour or more
- **Pain management:** fentanyl (0.5–1.5 mcg/kg/dose IV or intranasal), morphine (0.1 mg/kg/dose IV or IM), toradol (0.5 mg/kg IV to a maximum of 15 mg)
- **Labs:** CBC with diff, chem panel, UA, urine myoglobin (suspected muscle injury), carboxyhemoglobin level (suspected inhalation injury), ABG
- **Burn care:** cover with a dry sterile dressing pending transfer to a burn center. Avoid wet dressings that exacerbate hypothermia
- **Imaging:** dictated by the presence of concomitant injury
- **Monitor for rhabdomyolysis**
- Myalgias
- Generalized weakness
- Darkened urine

Minor Burns

- **Pain management:** options vary widely based on extent of burn injury and patient condition and comorbidities. Fentanyl 1 to 2 mcg/kg for severe injuries, hydromorphone 0.5 to 2 mg, morphine 2 to 10 mg. Acetaminophen and ibuprofen are also very effective in conjunction with opiates
- **Burn care:** clean burns with mild soap and water; debride devitalized tissue; leave blisters intact; avoid ice or prolonged soaking; apply a simple antibiotic ointment (e.g., bacitracin, Silvadene), or apply a commercially prepared synthetic occlusive dressing; cover with nonadherent dressing and wrap with woven gauze bandage

---

CRITERIA FOR ADMISSION TO A BURN CENTER:

- Partial thickness burns >20% TBSA at any age
- Full thickness burns >5% TBSA
- Any significant burn to the face, hands, joints, genitalia, or perineum
- Inhalation, chemical, or electrical injury
- Significant associated injuries
- **Pts who do not meet these criteria should be admitted to an inpt burn unit if any of the following are present:**
- Age >10 with >10% TBSA affected
- Inability to take PO fluids, full thickness burns
- 2% TBSA; high voltage injuries, circumferential burns; suspected maltreatment

(cont.)

BURNS (cont.)

DICTATION/DOCUMENTATION

- **General:** awake and alert, not toxic appearing
- **VS and SaO$_2$**
- **Skin:** estimated % TBSA of burn and method of calculation (e.g., Lund and Browder chart); depth and description of burns; presence of circumferential burns
- **HEENT:**
  - **Head:** atraumatic, nontender
  - **Eyes:** sclera and conjunctiva clear, PERRLA, EOMI
  - **Ears:** TMs and canals clear
  - **Nose/Face:** no facial burn, nasal flare
  - **Mouth/Throat:** lips without burns or STS, no drooling, stridor, dysphagia, odor of soot on breath, carbonaceous secretions, intraoral burns MMM, posterior pharynx clear, voice normal
- **Neck:** supple, FROM, no STS
- **Chest:** no surface burn, no retractions or accessory muscle use; CTA, no wheezing, rhonchi, crackles
- **Heart:** RRR, no murmurs, rubs, or gallops
- **Abd:** no surface burn, soft, BSA, NT
- **Extrems:** no surface burns, STS, FROM, good muscle strength and tone, pulses intact in all limbs

⊙ TIP

- Palmar surface of the patient's hand = ~1% of TBSA

HEADACHE

HX

- Onset: first HA, sudden onset or change from normal HA
- "Worst ever," "thunderclap," "throbbing"
- Alleviating factors: light, sound, position, foods
- Duration, quality, radiation, unilateral or bilateral, frequency, time of day F/C, N/V
- Vision: blurred, photophobia, diplopia, loss of vision, lines, spots
- Nasal congestion, sinus pain, cough, dental problem
- Decreased or loss of hearing, tinnitus
- Facial or temporal tenderness, facial asymmetry
- Neck pain, stiffness
- Dizziness, fainting, seizure
- Muscle weakness, numbness, tingling, problems with balance or speech
- Worse in a.m. (carbon monoxide)
- Rash
- LNMP
- Recent trauma, onset after exertion
- Changes in medication; medication withdrawal
- PMH: HTN, CVA, cardiac, FH of HA

PE

- **General:** alert, not toxic appearing
- **VS:** fever
- **Skin:** PWD, rash, petechiae
- **HEENT:**
  - **Head:** trigger point, scalp tenderness
  - **Eyes:** PERRLA, sclera, conjunctiva, corneas, EOMI, fundi. Note nystagmus, diplopia, ptosis, tearing, conjunctival injection, IOP if measured
  - **Ears:** canals and TMs
  - **Nose:** drainage, congestion
  - **Face:** sinus tenderness, facial swelling, decreased pulsation or tenderness over temple, TMJ tenderness
  - **Mouth/Throat:** MMM, condition of teeth
- **Neck:** supple, FROM, lymphadenopathy, meningismus
- **Chest:** CTA
- **Abd:** soft, NT
- **Extremities:** moves all extremities with good strength, distal motor/sensory intact, good pulses
- **Neuro:** A&O × 4, GCS, CN II–XII, focal neuro deficit, DTRs, pathological reflexes, speech/gait, Romberg, pronator drift, speech clear, gait steady

(cont.)

HEADACHE (cont.)

MDM/DDx

In general, older adults experience fewer episodes of headache compared to younger pts and the etiology may be life-threatening. The MDM must include consideration of more serious primary or secondary causes of headache. Careful consideration of **transient cerebral ischemia, cerebrovascular disease, subarachnoid hemorrhage, acute narrow angle closure glaucoma, giant cell arteritis,** or infectious causes, such as **meningitis or encephalitis,** is essential. Differential diagnoses of less serious headaches in the older adult includes **cluster** or **tension headaches and migraines. Late-life migraines** often present with visual or sensory changes or awaken the pt from sleep. Long-standing migraines usually decrease in incidence as people age. **Hypnic headaches** are rare and usually affect people over 60 years of age, who awaken from sleep with a throbbing headache. Other causes of headache to investigate include **sinus** or **dental infection, trigeminal neuralgia, herpes zoster, TMJ problems,** or **medication withdrawal.**

MANAGEMENT

- Minimize visual and auditory stimuli, cold compresses, antiemetic
- IV NS 1 L often helpful. Older adults may need fluid restriction if comorbidities (e.g., CHF)
- Analgesia options vary widely
- Acetaminophen is the safest drug for symptomatic treatment of migraine in older adults. NSAIDs *may cause GI bleeding and opioids can lead to confusion or sedation.* For acute management, prochlorperazine 5 to 10 mg IV or promethazine 25 mg IV plus diphenhydramine 25 mg IV (limit use in the older adult); metoclopramide 10 to 20 mg IV; abortive agents, such as triptans, may be effective; opioids, such as dilaudid 1 to 2 mg IV, in severe cases *(lower dose in the older adult)*
- Older adults can use topiramate, metoprolol, and propranolol for migraine prevention. Low-dose antidepressants are well tolerated and effective in the older adult. Botulinum toxin type A may be effective for failed alternative treatments. Hypnic headaches may respond to caffeine, lithium, or verapamil.
- Avoid amitriptyline and doxepin in older adults because of possible cognitive impairment, urinary retention, or cardiac arrhythmia
- Imaging not usually needed with HX migraine and normal neuro exam
- Admit for intractable N/V or pain
  - Cluster HA may respond to 100% O_2 6 to 8 L/min via nonrebreather mask if started at onset of HA

(cont.)

HEADACHE (cont.)

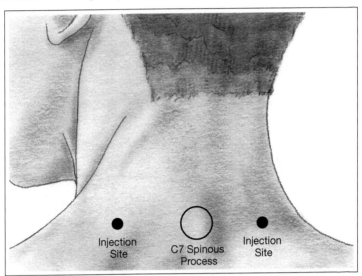

Injection Site

C7 Spinous Process

Injection Site

Lower paracervical intramuscular injection sites

LOWER PARACERVICAL INTRAMUSCULAR INJECTION PROCEDURE NOTE

Procedure explained and consent obtained. Pt was placed in a seated position and the posterior seventh cervical vertebrae landmark palpated. Sterile drape and prep was done and injection sites were located 2 to 3 cm lateral to the spinous process. A 25 or 27 gauge needle was introduced 1 to 1.5 inches parallel to the top of the shoulder in a posterior to anterior direction. Bupivacaine 1.5 mL was slowly injected into the lower paraspinous muscle. The needle was withdrawn and the area massaged to promote absorption of the medication. DSD was applied. Lung sounds were CTA bilaterally after the procedure and the pt tolerated the procedure well. Pain level was ___/0–10 post procedure. Tolerated procedure well without complications.

(cont.)

HEADACHE (cont.)

CRANIAL NERVES

I	Olfactory	Sense of smell
II	Optic	Visual acuity, visual fields, fundi
III	Oculomotor	Pupillary function, EOM function of IO, SR, MR, IR
IV	Trochlear	EOM function of SO
V	Trigeminal	Facial sensation to light touch, temperature, facial muscle strength, corneal reflex
VI	Abducens	EOM function of LR
VII	Facial	Symmetry of facial expressions (e.g., smile, frown, wrinkle forehead), taste anterior 2/3 of the tongue
VIII	Acoustic	Whisper test, tuning fork lateralization
IX	Glossopharyngeal	Gag reflex, swallow, taste posterior 1/3 of tongue
X	Vagus	Gag reflex, swallow, hoarseness, soft palate sensation
XI	Spinal accessory	Shoulder shrug and turn head against resistance
XII	Hypoglossal	Tongue symmetry, movement, strength

DICTATION/DOCUMENTATION

- **General:** awake and alert, not toxic appearing
- **VS:** no fever or tachycardia
- **SaO$_2$:** WNL
- **Skin:** PWD, no lesions or rash, no petechiae
- **HEENT:**
    - **Head:** scalp atraumatic, NT, no trigger points
    - **Eyes:** sclera and conjunctiva clear, corneas grossly clear, PERRLA, EOMI, no nystagmus, no ptosis, no photophobia, normal funduscopic exam, normal visual fields, IOP
    - **Ears:** canals and TMs normal. Nose/Face: no rhinorrhea, congestion; no frontal or maxillary sinus TTP; no asymmetry
    - **Mouth/Throat:** MMM, no erythema or exudate
- **Neck:** supple, FROM, NT, no lymphadenopathy, no meningismus
- **Chest:** CTA
- **Heart:** RRR, no murmurs, rubs, or gallops
- **Extremities:** moves all extremities with good strength, normal gait
- **Neuro:** A&O × 4; GCS 15; CN II–XII grossly intact. No focal neurological deficits. Normal muscle strength and tone. Normal DTRs, negative Babinski, normal finger-to-nose coordination or heel-to-shin glide. Speech clear, normal gait. Negative Romberg, no pronator drift

(cont.)

HEADACHE (cont.)

⊙ TIPS

- New-onset migraines are unusual in older adults and migraine incidence decreases with age
- Consider occult or subacute subdural hematoma as headache cause
- Trigeminal neuralgia occurs most commonly in older adults
- Cervical spondylosis can cause secondary headache in older adults
- Always proceed with caution in the management of a headache in a pt who is on an anticoagulant

DON'T MISS!

- Other causes of headache: structural, infectious, or metabolic etiologies

DIZZY/WEAK

HX

- Onset, intensity, and duration are important clues
- Positional, exacerbated by movement of neck or head
- False sense of motion: feeling of room spinning or pt spinning
- Feeling off balance, about to fall or faint, light-headed, disoriented
- Headache, N/V, sweating
- Visual changes, blurred vision, loss of vision
- Loss of hearing/tinnitus, ear pain, or fullness (peripheral causes)
- Antalgic or ataxia gait; increased falls
- Numbness, tingling, focal weakness
- Vomiting blood, or blood in stool, trauma
- Fever, poor fluid intake
- CP/dysrhythmias, SOB, syncope, seizure
- Hypoglycemia/hyperglycemia or hyponatremia/hypernatremia
- Illicit drugs/ETOH/smoking
- Medication HX: antihypertensives, antiarrhythmics, antianxiolytics for situational anxiety/hyperventilation

PE

- **General:** mental status, able to walk or sit up with normal trunk strength
- **VS and SaO$_2$:** tachycardia, bradycardia, dysrhythmias, orthostatic changes
- **Skin:** pale, cool, moist, hot, flushed
- **HEENT:**
  - **Head:** normocephalic, atraumatic
  - **Eyes:** PERRLA, EOMI, ptosis. Changes in gaze. Nystagmus or rhythmic oscillation of eye. Vertical (central), unidirectional with fixed gaze or rotational (peripheral), horizontal (possible ETOH), BPPV occurs with the head in a specific position
  - **Ears:** canals and TMs normal, vesicles, hearing
  - **Nose:** normal
  - **Face:** symmetry, facial droop, sensation to light touch and temperature
  - **Mouth/Throat:** MMM, posterior pharynx clear
- **Neck:** supple, FROM, no lymphadenopathy or meningismus
- **Chest:** CTA
- **Abd:** soft, BSA, NT
- **Back:** spinal or CVAT
- **Extremities:** FROM with good strength, distal motor/sensory intact, good pulses
- **Neuro:** A&O × 4, GCS 15, CN I–XII intact, no focal neuro deficits, normal finger-to-nose or heel-to-shin testing, Romberg neg, no pronator drift, rapid alternating movements. Gait is normal, cautious, wide-based, ataxic, tandem gait with eyes closed

(cont.)

DIZZY/WEAK (cont.)

MDM/DDx

Weakness: it is important to distinguish between weakness and fatigue in older adults. Weakness can be either focal or generalized. Unilateral focal weakness is often caused by **stroke**; other causes include **neuropathies, nerve root entrapment,** or **spinal cord compression.** Causes of generalized weakness include **frailty of old age, inactivity,** or **immobilization.** Many **serious** and **chronic diseases** can cause fatigue or exhaustion in the older adult. Consider **malignancy, infection, heart failure, COPD, anemia, renal/hepatic failure, electrolyte derangement, hypothyroidism,** or **anemia.** Many older pts also have **depression** and some have **fibromyalgia or chronic fatigue syndrome,** but a diligent search for undetected causes of fatigue must be conducted. **Dizziness:** dizziness is a common and debilitating problem for older adults. The vestibular system ages and functions less efficiently; preexisting medical problems, such as **stroke, peripheral neuropathy,** visual impairment, and immobility, make dizziness a serious concern in the older adult. Several other causes of dizziness in the older adult must also be considered. Although most often caused by a **peripheral vestibular origin** (ear), older pts must be evaluated for more serious causes of dizziness such as **CNS dysfunction.** This group is also at higher risk **for cardiovascular problems, metabolic derangement, infection, dehydration,** and medication-related problems that can present with dizziness. The older adults are less likely to have dizziness of a psychogenic nature compared to younger people. **Vertigo:** all vertigo is affected but not provoked by head movement. Very brief episodes of vertigo *associated with rapid head movement* suggest **benign paroxysmal positional vertigo is very common in older adults who** complain of dizziness and vertigo that is worsened by movement of the head or getting out of bed. **Meniere's disease** is also common in older adults and produces prolonged symptoms for hours of severe vertigo, "roaring" tinnitus, a feeling of ear fullness or pressure, and decreased hearing. Dizziness with hearing loss and recent viral illness may be caused by **labyrinthitis. Abrupt onset of** vertigo lasting days to weeks and associated with N/V, ataxia, and nystagmus without hearing changes or neurological findings suggests **vestibular neuronitis.** Ototoxic medications, such as gentamicin, furosemide, and some NSAIDs, can cause hearing loss and balance issues. Diplopia, dysarthria, dysphagia, motor and sensory changes, or syncope are serious findings that may be caused by **brainstem ischemia** or **multiple sclerosis.** Light-headedness and imbalance on assuming upright posture may be the result of orthostatic **changes** caused by antihypertensive or antiarrhythmic medications. Vertigo lasting minutes to hours with hearing changes and headache is often **migrainous** in origin but is less common as one ages. Vague "heavy-headedness," light-headedness, and feeling "off balance" without true vertigo and lack of physical findings may be related to **anxiety** disorders but often require neuro referral to rule out serious causes. Rarely, nonmalignant tumors of the eighth CN (acoustic neuroma) can cause dizziness and hearing loss. Sudden, severe weakness/dizziness with chest pain radiating to the back may indicate **MI, ACS, CAD, AAA, TAD, or PE. Seizures** are an uncommon cause of dizziness or very brief sensation of spinning or loss of consciousness.

MANAGEMENT

- **Central vertigo:** basic labs, EKG + CT/MRI or CT-A, neuro consult
- **Peripheral vertigo:** meclizine 25 mg QID—use with caution in older adults because of side effects. Antiemetics. HCTZ for Meniere's disease
- **Weak/light-headed/syncope:** EKG, IV volume replacement, monitor, basic labs with cardiac enzymes, coags, T&S, CT/MRI as indicated; possible cardiac or neuro consult; likely admit
- Specialty consultation and referral to neurology, cardiology, or ENT as indicated. Older adults may benefit from vestibular physical therapy

(cont.)

DIZZY/WEAK (cont.)

DICTATION/DOCUMENTATION

- **General:** alert and active. Ambulates to treatment area with normal gait
- **VS and SaO$_2$:** normal, no orthostatic changes
- **Skin:** PWD, no pallor
- **HEENT:**
  - **Head:** normocephalic, atraumatic
  - **Eyes:** PERRLA, conjunctivae pink, EOMI, no ptosis or nystagmus
  - **Ears:** canals and TMs normal, no vesicles, hearing normal
  - **Nose:** normal
  - **Face:** no facial asymmetry, sensation to light, touch and temperature intact and symmetrical
  - **Mouth/Throat:** MMM, normal rise of soft palate, posterior pharynx clear
- **Neck:** supple, FROM, no lymphadenopathy or meningismus
- **Chest:** CTA
- **Heart:** RRR, no murmurs, rubs, or gallops
- **Abd:** soft, +BSA, NT
- **Rectal:** brown stool, OB negative
- **Back:** no spinal or CVAT
- **Extrems:** FROM with good strength, distal motor/sensory intact and symmetrical, good pulses
- **Neuro:** A&O × 4, GCS 15, CN I–XII intact, no focal neuro deficits, normal finger-to-nose or heel-to-shin testing, Romberg neg, no pronator drift, normal rapid alternating movements. Gait is normal, cautious, wide-based, and ataxic; tandem gait with eyes closed

◯ TIPS

- **Dizziness:** sense of lightheadedness or disorientation
- **True vertigo:** feeling that environment is rotating or spinning, often associated with nausea
- **Central vertigo:** brainstem or cerebellum—diplopia, N/V, trouble with speech or swallowing, focal weakness, ataxia or unable to ambulate, sudden spontaneous fall with rapid recovery
- **Peripheral vertigo:** inner ear or vestibular nerve—awake and alert, N/V, usually able to ambulate, very brief episodes of vertigo associated with rapid head movement, tinnitus or hearing loss, HX migraine, recent upper respiratory infection (URI), or barotrauma

DON'T MISS!

- New change in LOC
- Focal neurological deficit
- Symptoms lasting over 1 hour
- Difficulty with ambulation/ataxia
- Head or neck pain
- Presentation with concern for CVA

ALTERED MENTAL STATUS

AMS is a significant presenting problem in older adult pts. There is no "classic presentation." **The most broadly accepted classifications of AMS are delirium, dementia, and psychosis** with different causes and treatments. Identification of potential causes is essential. Most common etiologies are:

- Neurological problems
- Infections
- Metabolic derangement

HX

Onset/Duration/Characteristics

- Delirium (usually more rapid—fluctuates, visual hallucinations)
- Dementia (usually more gradual—progressive, no hallucinations, changes in social interaction, crying/repetitive vocalization, hypersexuality, sleep disturbances, inappropriate dressing/disrobing, physical aggression, changes in ability to perform basic ADLs, substance abuse. Psychosis (variable, may have auditory hallucinations)

Other HX Questions

- Note if pt is "poor historian"
- Decreased PO fluid intake/dehydration, polyuria, polydipsia
- Trauma: recent or HX TBI (risk for dementia)
- Recent falls or inc falling (more likely with dementia)
- Ingestion/drug OD/ETOH; carbon monoxide or toxin exposure
- New or recently changed/stopped meds, OTC, home remedies, antihypertensive, anticoagulants, opioids, benzodiazepines, antiepileptic
- F/C, N/V, D/C
- Hypoglycemia, sweating
- HA, neck pain or stiffness, dizziness/syncope/vertigo/seizure
- Visual changes, blurred vision, loss of vision
- Loss of hearing/tinnitus, ear pain
- Changes in speech—dysarthria or aphasia/vision—diplopia/memory (Mini-Cognitive)
- CP/dysrhythmia, SOB
- Weakness, tremors, bowel/bladder function, melena

PMH

- Cardiac and/or cerebrovascular disease
- Renal/Meta: DM, DKA/HHS, CRF, hypo/hypernatremia
- Endo: thyroid, Addison's disease
- Neuro: HA, SAH, seizure, tremors (e.g., Parkinson's), dementia, numbness, tingling, focal weakness; antalgic or ataxia gait, balance problems, motor/sensory changes
- Psych: anxiety/hyperventilation, major depressive disorder
- Immunosuppressed: CA, HIV

(cont.)

ALTERED MENTAL STATUS (cont.)

PE

- **General:** alert, disoriented, confused, tremulous, arousable, agitated, lethargic, stuporous, delirious, comatose. Recognition/interaction with family members or significant others
- **Hygiene:** trauma; odors (ETOH, acetone, almonds)
- **LOC:** delirium altered; dementia normal; psychosis variable
- **VS and SaO$_2$:** fever/hypothermia, brady/tachycardia, resp depression, hypo/hyperventilation
- **Skin:** texture, turgor, rash, petechiae/purpura, jaundice, needle marks
- **HEENT:**
  - **Head:** surface trauma
  - **Eyes:** PERRLA, fixed/dilated, icterus, EOMI, ptosis, fundi (papilledema, retinal hemorrhage)
  - **Ears:** canals patent, hemotympanum, CSF leak
  - **Nose:** CSF leak
  - **Face:** symmetric, weakness
  - **Mouth/Throat:** gag reflex, tongue symmetry
- **Neck:** meningismus, nuchal rigidity, thyroid
- **Chest:** CTA
- **Heart:** RRR, resp effort
- **Abd:** soft, NT, pulsatile mass, ascites, hepatomegaly, suprapubic TTP or distension
- **Back:** no evidence of trauma, no spinal or CVAT
- **Rectal:** tone, occult blood, melena
- **Extremities:** FROM, NT, strength and sensation, weakness, tremors, asterixis (liver hand flap), rigidity
- **Neuro:** A&O × 4, GCS 15, CN II–XII, focal neuro deficit, DTRs, pathological reflexes, speech/gait, Romberg, pronator drift, speech clear, gait steady, spontaneous or uncontrolled movements, abnormal posturing, flaccid

MDM/DDx

Pts with AMS can present with a range of SXS from slightly confused to comatose. A thorough HX, knowledge of a pts baseline, and comprehensive physical exam are essential. **AMS is not a diagnosis and often there are multiple diagnoses involved.** Initial efforts are directed toward stabilization of ABCs, evaluation for a critical illness/injury, and admission/transfer to an appropriate facility (e.g., psychiatric). Causes of AMS include neurological dysfunction, metabolic derangement, infection, toxin, or psychiatric etiologies. Cognitive function is normal in schizophrenia or affective/bipolar disorders but abnormal if psychosis is caused by an underlying disease or structural problems. **Hypoxia and hypoglycemia, opiate ingestion, intracranial hemorrhage,** and UTI are some of the causes of **delirium** that should be identified and treated. **Head trauma** may or may not be evident, so a high index of suspicion is warranted. Assess for signs of **infection** such as hypo/hyperthermia and tachycardia, nuchal rigidity, and/or petechiae. **Urosepsis** and **pneumonia** are common infections that cause delirium. Immediate Abx should be administered for pts if **sepsis** is suspected. For delirium of unclear etiology consider **Alzheimer's disease, vascular dementia, Lewy-body dementia,** or **frontotemporal dementia**

(cont.)

ALTERED MENTAL STATUS (cont.)

MANAGEMENT

- Identify pt's baseline cognitive function (HX from the family, caretakers)
- Identify and treat reversible causes:
  - Severe pain
  - Infection
  - Dehydration
  - Electrolyte imbalance
  - Hypoxia
  - Elimination problems
  - Sensory deprivation
- R/O depression (see "Geriatric Depression Scale")
- Maintain behavioral control by placing the pt in a safe and quiet environment under constant surveillance; provide simple instructions and explanations
- ABCs (with spinal protection if trauma suspected)
- O_2, IV NS; volume replacement if dehydrated, hypotensive, or concern for HHS
- FSBS, CBC, chem panel, UA, Utox
- EKG, CXR
- Consider: LFTs, ABG, specific drug levels, ETOH, ammonia level, cortisol level, carboxyhemoglobin
- Head CT, LP, C-spine x-ray (if trauma)
- Correct electrolyte imbalance
- Rewarming/cooling measures for hypo/hyperthermia

Causes/Treatment

- **Hypoglycemia**: dextrose
- **Opioid toxicity:** Narcan
- **Infection:** Abx for suspected infection
- **Thiamine:** if indicated (e.g., alcoholism)
- **Hypertensive encephalopathy:** anti-HTN agents (e.g., labetalol, nitroprusside)
- **Toxins:** specific antidotes as needed
- **Agitation:** PRN options, monitor for side effects of sedation and respiratory depression
  - Haloperidol: 0.25 to 1 mg PO, IM or IV q4h (monitor for prolonged QT)
  - Olanzapine: 2.5 to 5 mg PO or IM q12h. Max dose 20 mg in 24 hours
  - Lorazepam: 0.25 to 1 mg PO or IV q8h; risperidone: 0.25 to 1 mg PO q4h; quetiapine: 25 to 50 mg PO q12h
- **Manic-like behaviors:** Depakote 125 mg q12h, slowly titrate monitoring for side effects; lamotrigine 25 to 200 mg/d
- Antidepressants
  - **Disturbance of sleep cycle:** mirtazapine 7.5 mg starting dose; trazodone 25 to 50 mg starting dose. Prepare for acute hospital, psychiatric facility admission, or care facility placement; consults as indicated

(cont.)

ALTERED MENTAL STATUS (cont.)

DICTATION/DOCUMENTATION

- **General:** agitated, noncooperative; LOC, CAM. Assessment results; describe current behavior; not toxic appearing; no odors
- **VS and SaO$_2$:** VSS, no fever, tachycardia, or hypoxemia
- **Skin:** PWD, no lesions, rash, or surface trauma noted
- **HEENT:**
    - **Head:** atraumatic, NT
    - **Eyes:** sclera and conjunctiva clear, corneas grossly clear, PERRLA, EOMI, no nystagmus, disconjugate gaze, or ptosis. Corneal reflex intact. Funduscopic exam WNL
    - **Ears:** canals and TMs normal. No hemotympanum or Battle's sign
    - **Nose/Face:** atraumatic, NT, no asymmetry
    - **Mouth/Throat:** MMM, posterior pharynx clear, normal gag reflex, no intraoral trauma
- **Neck:** supple, FROM, NT, no lymphadenopathy, no meningismus
- **Chest:** CTA, no wheezes, rhonchi, rales. Normal TV, no retractions or accessory muscle use. No respiratory depression
- **Heart:** RRR, no murmurs, rubs, or gallops
- **Abd:** soft, NT, no pulsatile mass, ascites, hepatosplenomegaly, suprapubic TTP or distension
- **Back:** without spinal or CVA tenderness
- **Extrems:** FROM with good strength, distal motor neurovascular intact
- **Neuro:** A&O × 4, GCS 15, CN II–XII grossly intact. No focal neuro deficits. Normal muscle strength and tone. Normal DTRs, negative Babinski, normal finger-to-nose coordination or heel-to-shin glide. Speech, gait, Romberg neg, no pronator drift

CONFUSION ASSESSMENT METHOD

- Diagnosis of **delirium** requires *both:*
- Acute change in mental status and fluctuating course
- Inattention, and difficulty focusing attention
    and *either:*
    - Disorganized thinking
    - Altered level of consciousness (anything other than alert)

◉ TIPS

- AMS is not part of the normal aging process—look for underlying cause
- FSBS and UA dip are rapid tests to evaluate for common causes of AMS

DON'T MISS!

- CVA
- Drug overdose
- Medication reaction
- Depression
- Alcoholism

ACTIVITIES OF DAILY LIVING

- Bathing
- Dressing
- Feeding
- Toileting
- Transferring
- Continence
- Managing money
- Use of communication devices
- Shopping
- Preparing food
- Housekeeping
- Laundry
- Transportation (able to drive)
- Managing medications

MENTAL STATUS EXAM

- **General Behavior**
  - Mood and affect
  - Insight and judgment
  - Thought and language → psychotic
  - Cognitive function → organic
- **Thought and Language**
  - Thought process
  - Connections between thoughts
  - Thought content
  - The actual thoughts (delusions, etc.)
  - Perception
  - Misinterpretation of real objects (illusions)
  - Hallucinations
- **Abnormal Perception**
  - Hallucinations
  - Auditory
  - Most common in schizophrenia: visual, gustatory, olfactory, tactile. Assume medical cause till proven otherwise
- **Etiologies of Acute Organic Brain Syndromes**
  - Organic brain syndrome—behavioral disorder with a "nonpsychiatric" medical/surgical cause
  - Toxic
    - Prescribed or abused drugs
    - Side effect, intoxication, or withdrawal
    - Toxins
    - Plants, poisons
  - Infection
    - Brain
    - Encephalitis, meningitis
    - Any other organ
    - Systemi
  - Neurosurgical
    - Occult subdural hematoma
    - Concussion
    - Traumatic brain injury
    - Abscess
    - Tumor
  - Neurologic
    - Postictal
    - Degenerative
    - Alzheimer's, multi-infarct, and so on
    - Various encephalopathies
  - Cerebrovascular
    - Stroke
    - TIA
    - Multi-infarct dementia
    - Vasculitis
    - Hypotension

(cont.)

MENTAL STATUS EXAM (cont.)

- Metabolic
  - Glucose
  - Electrolytes
  - Hypoxia
  - Hepatic failure
  - Renal failure
- Endocrine
  - Thyroid
  - Parathyroid
  - Adrenal
  - Pituitary
- Oncologic
  - Brain
  - Systemic
  - Hormone secreting tumor
- **Life-Threatening Psychiatric Conditions**
  - Suicidal ideation
  - Homicidal ideation
  - Grave mental disability
  - Involuntary psychiatric holds

HEAD INJURY

HX

- Time on injury, MOI (auto vs. ped, ejection, significant fall)
- ALOC: gradual, sudden LOC, brief lucid interval
- HA, visual changes, seizure
- Blood/CSF leak nose/ears
- Neck/back pain, N/V
- Age >60, use of anticoags, ETOH
- Distracting injury, suspected open or depressed skull FX

PE

- **General:** position of pt (full spinal precautions)
- **VS and SaO$_2$:** tachycardia or bradycardia (significant for shock/neurogenic shock), widening pulse pressure
- **Skin:** warm, dry, cool, moist, pale
- **HEENT:**
    - **Head:** surface trauma, TTP, bony step-off
    - **Eyes:** PERRLA, EOMI, periorbital ecchymosis
    - **Ears:** canals patent, TMs, Battle's sign, hemotympanum, CSF leak
    - **Nose:** nasal injury, septal hematoma, epistaxis, CSF rhinorrhea
    - **Face:** facial trauma
    - **Mouth/Throat:** intraoral trauma, teeth and mandible stable
- **Neck:** FROM without limitation or pain, NT to firm palp at midline
- **Chest:** NT, CTA
- **Heart:** RRR, no murmurs, rubs, or gallops.
- **Abd:** BSA, NT
- **Back:** no spinal or CVAT
- **Pelvis:** NT to palpation and stable to compression, femoral pulses strong and equal
- **Extremities:** FROM, NT, distal CMS intact
- **Neuro:** A&O × 4, GCS 15, no focal neuro deficits

CONCUSSION ASSESSMENT CRITERIA:

- Recall of person, place, time, events?
- Five simple word recall
- Months of year in reverse order
- Random three to six numbers in reverse: if able to recall three digits correctly in reverse order, increase number of digits in sequence, speech, pupils, EOMs, gait

Source: Adapted from McCroy, P., Johnson, K., Meeuwisse, W., Aubry, M., Cantu, R., Dvorak, J., ... Schamasch, P. (2005). Summary and agreement statement of the 2nd International Conference on Concussion in Sport, Prague 2004. *British Journal of Sports Medicine, 39*(4), 196–204. doi:10.1136/bjsm.2005.018614

(cont.)

HEAD INJURY (cont.)

MDM/DDx

People older than 65 years are at significant risk for **traumatic brain injury** even from minor trauma. Older adults are much more likely to be hospitalized for **head injury** and have generally poorer outcomes and increased injury-related mortality. Falls account for over half of TBI in this age group but the exact mechanism of injury is often unknown. MDM must address preinjury functional level, comorbidities, risk prediction, and at-home support. Differential diagnoses considered include **mild blunt head injury** and/or **scalp laceration.** Serious problems include **concussion, skull fracture, subdural** or **epidural hematoma, cerebral contusion,** and **intracranial hemorrhage.** Also consider those pts with **high risk** for significant injury, drug/ETOH use, possible suicide attempt, distracting injuries, or anticoag use. Also, age >60 years, suspected open or depressed skull FX, evidence of basilar skull FX (periorbital ecchymosis, hemotympanum, Battle's sign, CSF leak), vomiting, GCS <15 at 2 hours postinjury, deteriorating during observation, or postinjury amnesia >2 to 4 hours. Consider **predictable injury** based on mechanism such as fall >3 ft or 5 stairs, ejection from vehicle, or auto versus pedestrian

MANAGEMENT

- Mild injury with low risk may be observed and given analgesia and antiemetic as needed; good ACI and close follow-up (F/U). Persistent N/V, severe headache, amnesia, LOC, or intoxication require head CT and observation of several hours before the decision to discharge. Consult neuro for abnormal CT findings or not stable for discharge

DICTATION/DOCUMENTATION

- **General:** awake and alert in no distress; no odor of ETOH
- **VS and SaO$_2$**
- **Skin:** PWD, no surface trauma
- **HEENT:**
  - **Head:** atraumatic, no palpable deformities
  - **Eyes:** PERRLA, EOMI, no periorbital ecchymosis
  - **Ears:** TMs clear, no hemotympanum or Battle's sign
  - **Nose/Face:** atraumatic. No septal hematoma. Facial bones symmetric, NT to palpation and stable with attempts at manipulation
  - **Mouth/Throat:** No intraoral trauma. Teeth and mandible are intact
- **Neck:** no point tenderness, step-off or deformity to firm palpation of the cervical spine at the midline. No spasm or paraspinal muscle tenderness. Trachea midline. Carotids equal. No masses. FROM without limitation or pain
- **Chest:** no surface trauma or asymmetry. NT without crepitus or deformity. Normal tidal volume. Breath sounds clear bilaterally. Oxygen saturation greater than 95% on room air
- **Heart:** RRR, no murmurs, rubs, or gallops. All peripheral pulses are intact and equal
- **Abd:** nondistended without abrasions or ecchymosis. BSA. No tenderness, guarding, or rebound. No masses. Good femoral pulses
- **Back:** no contusions, ecchymosis, or abrasions are noted. NT without step-off or deformity to firm palpation of the thoracic and lumbar spine
- **Pelvis:** NT to palpation and stable to compression
- **GU:** normal external genitalia with no blood at the meatus (if applicable)
- **Rectal:** normal tone. No rectal wall tenderness or mass. Stool is brown and heme negative (if applicable)
- **Extrems:** no surface trauma. FROM. Distal motor, neurovascular supply is intact
- **Neuro:** A&O × 4, GCS 15, CN II–XII grossly intact. Motor and sensory exam nonfocal. Reflexes are symmetric. Speech is clear and gait steady

(cont.)

HEAD INJURY (cont.)

DON'T MISS!

■ Anticoagulant use and falls

EYE PAIN

HX

- Baseline vision, previous HA or eye problems, surgeries, corrective glasses, contacts, or protective eyewear onset, duration, unilateral or bilateral visual changes: FB sensation, photophobia, diplopia, decreased or loss of vision, flashes of lights, halos, veil or curtain, scotoma (area of loss of vision surrounded by normal vision). Transient monocular blindness; consider AAA/TAD. Redness, discharge, tearing, itching, burning, swelling, painful or restricted eyeball movement. Nasal congestion, sinus pain, cough
- Facial lesions, redness, swelling, F/C, N/V, rash, genital lesions
- MOI: grinding metal or FB under pressure, chemical exposure, organic matter injury, blunt or penetrating trauma comorbidities
- HAs, migraines, DM, CAD, CA, HTN, glaucoma, macular degeneration, herpes sinus problems, ill contacts
- Eye surgery, cataract surgery with lens implant

PE

- **General:** level of distress
- **VS and SaO₂**
- **Skin:** warm dry, cool, moist, pale
- **HEENT:**
  - **Head:** surface trauma, TTP, bony step-off
  - **Eyes: visual acuity (VA):** Snellen chart, count fingers (CF), hand motion (HM), light or shadow or no light perception (NLP)
  - **Visual fields (VF):** full to confrontation (FTC)
  - **Periorbital:** STS, erythema, warmth, tenderness, bony step-off or deformity
  - **Eyelids:** erythema, crusting, swelling, FB/lesion on lid eversion, elevation (CN III); closure (CN VII)
  - **Eyeballs:** enophthalmos or exophthalmos, tenderness, intact
  - **Pupils:** PERRLA; CN II senses incoming light (afferent); CN III constricts pupil (efferent)
  - **Corneas:** grossly clear, steamy, no obvious FB or hyphema/hypopyon
  - **Sclera:** clear, injected, ciliary or limbic flush
  - **Conjunctiva:** palpebral and bulbar, subconjunctival hemorrhage, chemosis, evert lids
  - **EOMs intact:** symmetry of gaze, limitation or pain, nystagmus, ptosis, lid lag
  - **Lacrimal system:** canthus, papilla, puncta
  - **Funduscopic exam:** retina
  - **APD:** abn constriction due to unilateral afferent pathway problem
  - **Fluorescein stain exam:** corneal epithelial defect, abrasion, ulcer, dendritic lesion, FB, rust ring
  - **Slit lamp exam:** anterior chamber clear, or cell/flare, hyphema, hypopyon tonometry (Ta) measurement of IOP <20
  - **Ears:** canals and TMs, lesions
  - **Nose/Face:** drainage, congestion; TP, erythema, decreased pulsation of temporal artery, erythema, warmth, tenderness, bony step-off or deformity
  - **Mouth/Throat:** MMM, posterior pharynx
- **Neck:** supple, lymphadenopathy, meningismus

(cont.)

EYE PAIN (cont.)

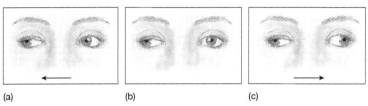

(a)   (b)   (c)

Right third nerve palsy examination (arrows indicate direction of gaze). Assessment findings include ptosis, ocular deviation (eye "down and out"), possible pupillary changes (fixed and dilated or loss of accommodation), diplopia.

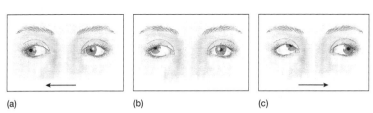

(a)   (b)   (c)

Right fourth nerve palsy examination (arrows indicate direction of gaze). Assessment findings include vertical or horizontal diplopia (especially looking down) when both eyes open and resolves when one eye covered, eye slightly "up and out", head tilt, possible supraorbital pain.

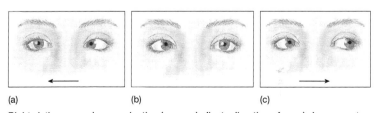

(a)   (b)   (c)

Right sixth nerve palsy examination (arrows indicate direction of gaze). Assessment findings include diplopia with lateral or distant gaze, eye slightly adducted with forward gaze, impaired abduction.

(cont.)

EYE PAIN (cont.)

MDM/DDx

Eye pain is a frequent complaint of older ED pts and can be divided into either ocular or orbital in nature. Ocular eye problems involve the structures of the surface of the eye and range from benign to vision-threatening problems. **Conjunctivitis** may be **allergic, viral, bacterial, fungal,** or **chemical** and can progress to involve the cornea (**keratitis** or **keratoconjunctivitis**), which may look like stippling or a punctate lesion. **A subconjunctival hemorrhage** is due to bleeding from the small blood vessels that run through the conjunctiva. The most common cause is idiopathic and the condition is painless and self-limiting; rarely, the redness may be associated with bleeding disorders (anticoags), conjunctivitis, scleritis, or trauma to the eye. **FBs** under the upper lid or embedded in the cornea are a common problem; **metallic FBs** can cause a rust ring and result in visual defects. Damage to the corneal epithelium leads to painful **corneal abrasions** that fluoresce under cobalt light. Fluorescein stain can also identify **dendritic lesions** caused by HSV. HZV can cause a **pseudodendrite** and may be associated with facial HZV lesions; **Hutchinson's sign** is an HZV lesion on the tip of the nose that has a high correlation to involvement of the eye. Severe pain, tearing, blurred vision, and focal whitish infiltrate in stromal layer indicate a **corneal ulcer,** a common complication of contact lens use. This ophthalmologic emergency can lead to **permanent visual damage** and/or **perforation. Periorbital infections** include infections of the soft tissues or lacrimal system. **Periorbital cellulitis (referred to as preseptal)** involves the area anterior to the orbital septum, which acts as a barrier to the actual eyeball. The area is swollen, erythematous, and warm but movement of the EOMs is unlimited and painless and there is no proptosis. **Dacryocystitis** is an inflammation of the lacrimal duct or sac while **dacryoadenitis** involves the lacrimal gland in the supraorbital area. A **stye (hordeolum)** is a localized infection or inflammation of the eyelid margin involving hair follicles of the eyelashes (i.e., external hordeolum) or meibomian glands (i.e., internal hordeolum). A **chalazion** is a painless granuloma of the meibomian glands. **Orbital cellulitis** results when infection has spread to the eyeball itself. The pt appears ill with fever, visual changes, headache, and restricted and painful movement of the eye. Proptosis and possible meningeal signs may be present. **Orbital pain** results from eyeball disease or trauma and causes a deep ache in or behind the eye. Deeper structure problems include **iritis** and **uveitis** and are characterized by severe pain unrelieved by topical anesthesia, tearing, and ciliary or limbic flush. SLE will usually reveal cells and flare from inflammation. Nausea, vomiting, and headache are common complaints of pts with a painful red eye caused by **acute narrow-angle glaucoma** and require immediate consultation. Complaints of **loss of vision** without pain ("quiet eye") suggest **detached retina, central retinal artery occlusion, complete hyphema, vitreous hemorrhage,** or **optic neuritis.** FBs may enter the eye and lodge in the intraocular space. Assess for **globe integrity** if penetrating trauma is suspected. Signs of globe disruption can be subtle, such as Seidel sign (leakage of fluorescein stain), or obvious visible vitreous humor. Eye pain can also be related to **sinusitis, dental problems, or migraine HA**

(cont.)

EYE PAIN (cont.)

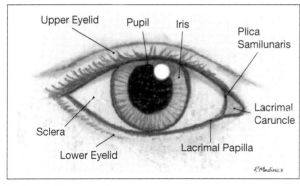

Upper Eyelid   Pupil   Iris   Plica Samilunaris

Lacrimal Caruncle

Sclera

Lower Eyelid   Lacrimal Papilla

Anatomy of the external eye

VISUAL FIELDS

- **Unilateral blindness:** (amaurosis fugax) transient loss of vision; TIA, optic neuritis, temporal arteritis
- **Bitemporal hemianopsia:** blindness of temporal or outer fields of both eyes; tumor
- **Homonymous hemianopsia:** optic tract problem causing blindness in temporal or nasal field of one or both eyes; stroke
- **Normal**
- **Unilateral field loss**
- **Bitemporal hemianopia**
- **Homonymous hemianopia**

APD "SWINGING LIGHT TEST": tests for light being "sensed" and needs intact pathway of globe, retina, and optic nerve. In a dark room, shine light into one eye; swing quickly to other, then back and forth. Normally, both pupils constrict equally without redilation. Affected pupil will not constrict if light not "sensed" but constricts when stimulated by light directed into normal eye, then dilates. Most common pupillary defect. Hyphema or vitreous hemorrhage will not cause APD

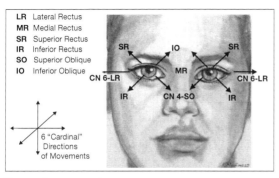

LR   Lateral Rectus
MR   Medial Rectus
SR   Superior Rectus
IR   Inferior Rectus
SO   Superior Oblique
IO   Inferior Oblique

SR   IO   SR
CN 6-LR   MR   CN 6-LR
IR   CN 4-SO   IR

6 "Cardinal" Directions of Movements

Extraocular movements

(cont.)

EYE PAIN (cont.)

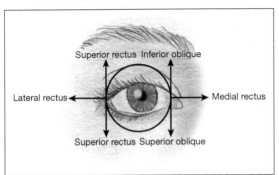

Eye muscles (right eye)

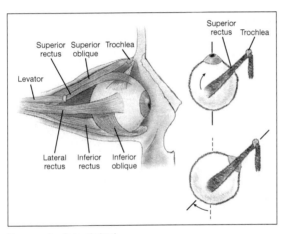

Eye muscles (lateral view)

(cont.)

EYE PAIN (cont.)

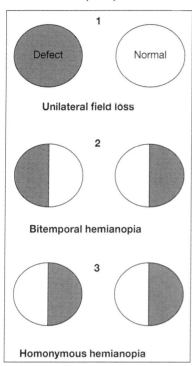

1
Defect   Normal

Unilateral field loss

2

Bitemporal hemianopia

3

Homonymous hemianopia

Visual field defects of the eye

(cont.)

EYE PAIN (cont.)

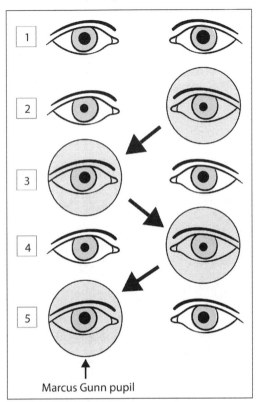

Marcus Gunn pupil

Diagram illustrating afferent pupillary defect (APD)
Source: Reproduced with permission from McGee, S. (2012).
Evidence-based physical diagnosis (3rd ed.). Philadelphia, PA:
Saunders.

(cont.)

EYE PAIN (cont.)

MANAGEMENT

- **Stye (Hordeolum):** warm soaks, NSAIDs, Abx for spread of infection, refer for possible drainage
- **Subconjunctival hemorrhage:** warm compresses may be useful in symptomatic relief. Treatment involves the identification and appropriate management of the underlying cause. Rarely, the redness may be associated with bleeding disorders (anticoags), conjunctivitis, scleritis, or trauma to the eye
- **Conjunctivitis/Keratitis:** usually viral, supportive care
- **Bacterial:** polymyxin B/trimethoprim 1 to 2 gtts every 3 to 6 hours × 7 to 10 days; erythromycin ointment ½" QID; levofloxacin 0.5% 1 to 2 gtts every 2 hours while awake × 2 days, then QID × 5 days; tobramycin 0.3% 1 to 2 gtts QID × 5 days
- **Contact lens:** ciprofloxacin 0.3% 1 to 2 gtts q1 to 6h; levofloxacin 0.5% gtts; tobramycin 0.3%–0.3% gtts; stop contact use. Recheck 1 day for corneal ulcer
- **Corneal FB:** topical anesthesia, tetanus status, removal with moistened cotton tip applicator, eye spud, sterile needle
- **Corneal abrasion:** topical/oral anesthesia, tetanus status, no patch, erythromycin ointment 1/2" QID; ciprofloxacin 0.3% 1 to 2 gtts; ofloxacin 1 to 2 gtts q1 to 6h
- **GC:** culture, ceftriaxone 1 g IM × 1. Admit pt for IV Rocephin
- **HSV:** topical/oral analgesia or cycloplegic gtts; trifluridine 1% gtts (max 9 gtts/d); acyclovir 800 mg PO five times a day × 7 to 10 days
- **Hyphema:** based on degree of hyphema. Topical/oral analgesia or cycloplegic gtts, topical/steroids, eye rest (bilateral patch), possible admit/surgery
- **HZV:** antivirals within 48 to 72 hours. Acyclovir 800 mg PO five times a day × 7 to 10 days (or valacyclovir, famciclovir)
- **Iritis/Uveitis:** oral analgesia and cycloplegic gtts; consult ophth for topical steroid use such as prednisolone 1% 1 to 2 gtts q1h initially
- **Orbital cellulitis:** fever control, analgesia, baseline labs, CT orbits and/or sinuses to R/O periorbital cellulitis; admit. Vancomycin 20 mg/kg BID plus ampicillin/sulbactam 3 g IV or clindamycin 600 to 900 mg IV TID, or piperacillin/tazobactam 4.5 g IV QID
- **Periorbital cellulitis:** outpt if nontoxic and F/U 1 day; admit <1 year or if severe; warm soaks, fever control, NSAIDs. CT orbits and/or sinuses to R/O cellulitis Abx (7–10 days): amoxicillin/clavulanate 875 PO BID; cephalexin 500 mg PO QID; clindamycin 300 to 450 PO TID; ampicillin/sulbactam 3 g IV, ceftriaxone 2 g IV; add vancomycin 20 mg/kg IV BID if MRSA
- **Narrow-angle glaucoma:** analgesia, antiemetic, place pt supine, consult ophth. Reduce IOP with acetazolamide 500 mg IV or PO plus topical beta-blocker, such as timolol 1 gtt BID, plus reduce inflammation with topical steroid such as prednisolone 1% 1 to 2 gtts. Possible miotic agent such as pilocarpine gtts and/or an osmotic, such as mannitol, may be used
- **Retinal detachment:** protect globe if traumatic; emergent ophthalmology referral

(cont.)

EYE PAIN (cont.)

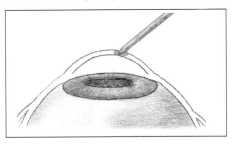
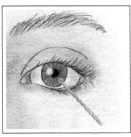

(a)   (b)

Superficial corneal foreign body removal

DICTATION/DOCUMENTATION

- **VA:** note whether corrective lenses used
- **Visual fields:** FTC
- **Medical**
  - No periorbital soft tissue swelling, erythema, or warmth. PERRLA. EOMI intact without limitation or complaint of pain. Lids and lashes clear. Sclera and conjunctiva are clear without erythema or exudates. No tearing or drainage. No ciliary flush. No chemosis. No photophobia. No lesions or rash of face or periocular area. Normal fundoscopic exam; no proptosis, enophthalmos, nystagmus. No APD. Note additional physical findings as indicated
- **Trauma**
  - No periorbital STS, ecchymosis, tenderness to palpation. No bony step-off or deformity. No palpable crepitus or subcutaneous air. PERRLA. EOMI without limitation or complaint of pain. No limitation in upward gaze. Corneal sensation normal. Sclera and conjunctiva are clear. No subconjunctival hemorrhage. No obvious foreign body or globe disruption. Corneas are grossly clear with no obvious hyphema

(cont.)

EYE PAIN (cont.)

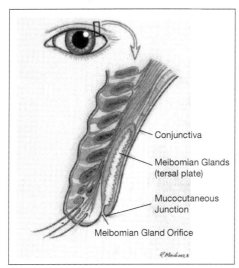

Conjunctiva

Meibomian Glands
(tersal plate)

Mucocutaneous
Junction

Meibomian Gland Orifice

Upper eyelid posterior anatomy

EARACHE

HX

- Onset, duration, F/C, N/V/D
- Nasal discharge, congestion, sinus pain
- Cough, sputum production
- Drainage, hearing loss
- HA
- Local trauma, exposure to water, foreign objects, day care
- Recent altitude changes, head injury
- Immunosuppressed, DM, HIV, atopic dermatitis, psoriasis, seborrheic dermatitis
- Hearing loss
- Use of hearing aids
- Impacted cerumen
- PMH: tinnitus, URIs, seasonal allergies
- Immunosuppressed HIV, DM, CA—evaluate for malignant otitis externa (*Pseudomonas aeruginosa*)
- Meds: previous use of ASA

PE

- **General:** alert, in no acute distress
- **VS and SaO$_2$:** fever, tachycardia, tachypnea
- **Skin:** PWD, normal texture and turgor; no lesions
- **HEENT:**
    - **Head:** NT
    - **Eyes:** PERRLA, EOMI, sclera and conjunctiva clear, drainage, periorbital STS, or erythema
    - **Ears:** Pre- or postauricular lymphadenopathy or erythema or lesions. Furuncle at external auditory meatus. Pain on movement of tragus or auricle, protrusion of auricle. Local swelling, scaling, eczematous skin. Canal: erythema, edema, exudate, FB. TM: erythema, bulging, retraction, landmarks, fluid level, bullae, perforation, cerumen
    - **Nose:** patent, NT, or hyperemic, rhinorrhea, edema
    - **Face:** facial asymmetry, loss of nasolabial fold, droop of mouth
    - **Mouth/Throat:** MMM, posterior pharynx clear, no erythema, exudate, vesicles, petechiae
- **Neck:** supple, NT, FROM, no meningismus or lymphadenopathy
- **Chest:** CTA or wheezes, rhonchi, rales, retractions
- **Abd:** soft, BSA, NT, no HSM
- **Back:** no spinal or CVAT
- **Neuro:** A&O × 4, GCS 15, no focal neuro deficits, normal behavior for age

(cont.)

EARACHE (cont.)

MDM/DDx

Evaluation of **ear pain (otalgia)** is directed toward determining whether the origin of pain is from the ear or referred from surrounding structures. Older adults, diabetics, and immunosuppressed pts should be evaluated for **malignant otitis externa**, most commonly caused by *Pseudomonas aeruginosa*. Ear pain can be caused by external otitis or otitis media, perforated TM, or infection of the outer ear. FB or cerumen impaction can also cause ear pain. Drainage from the ear canal should prompt consideration of **ruptured TM**. Prolonged episodes of otalgia with pain deep inside or behind the ear may indicate **acute mastoiditis**, a serious infection of the temporal bone associated with hearing loss and other complications. Older adults with otitis media should be evaluated for **pneumonia, dehydration,** or **sepsis. Dental, intraoral infections,** or **TMJ dysfunction** can present as acute ear pain

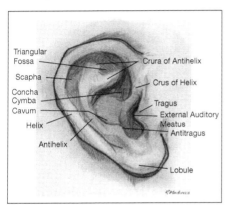

Ear anatomy

MANAGEMENT

- Pain fever control, NSAIDs
- **Otitis media:** usually viral
- **External otitis:** cerumen removal if indicated, acetic acid. Possible CT/MRI if severe. Abx: polymyxin B/neomycin/hydrocortisone 4 gtts QID; ofloxacin 0.3% sol 5 gtts BID; ciprofloxacin/-hydrocortisone 3 gtts BID or dicloxacillin 500 mg QID
- **Malignant otitis: consider antifungals in DM, HIV, chemo**. Abx: ciprofloxacin 750 mg BID × 6 weeks, or 400 mg IV TID; ceftazidime 2 g IV TID
  - Abx: (7–10 days): amoxicillin 45 mg/kg BID; PCN allergic: azithromycin 10 mg/kg × 1 day then 5 mg/kg × 4 days. If Abx in last month: amoxicillin/clavulanate 45 mg/kg BID
- **Mastoiditis:** possible CT/MRI and admission. Abx: ceftriaxone 50 mg/kg IV daily; clindamycin 7.5 mg/kg IV QID; vancomycin 15 to 20 mg/kg BID

(cont.)

EARACHE (cont.)

DICTATION/DOCUMENTATION

- **General:** awake and alert, not toxic appearing
- **VS and SaO$_2$:** (if indicated)
- **Skin:** PWD; no evidence of atopic dermatitis, psoriasis, seborrhea
- **HEENT:**
    - **Head:** atraumatic, NT; no scalp dermatitis
    - **Eyes:** sclera and conjunctiva clear, PERRLA, EOMI
    - **Ears:** no pre- or postauricular lymphadenopathy or erythema; canals are clear, no erythema, edema, exudates. No cerumen impaction. TMs normal without bulging or retraction. Good light reflex. No fluid level, vesicles, or bullae. No perforation
    - **Nose/Face:** no rhinorrhea, congestion; no frontal or maxillary sinus TTP
    - **Mouth/Throat:** MMM, posterior pharynx clear, no erythema or exudate
- **Neck:** supple, FROM, NT, no lymphadenopathy, no meningismus
- **Chest:** CTA

CERUMEN REMOVAL PROCEDURE NOTE

Procedure explained and consent obtained. The pt had cerumen removed from the L/R ear canal with a loop in order to visualize the tympanic membrane. Tolerated procedure well with no complications

---

▶ TIP

- Pts who take antibiotics for infection and who are taking Coumadin or warfarin need to have close monitoring of the INR before, during, and after antibiotic treatment. Important that the pt's PCP is notified about the addition of an antibiotic for the pt who is on an anticoagulant

DON'T MISS!

- Toxic appearing
- Unable to tolerate PO fluids; dehydration
- Meningismus
- Mastoiditis
- Malignant otitis externa
- Pneumonia

NASAL PAIN/INJURY

HX

- HA
- F/C
- MOI (trauma), circumstances
- LOC, N/V
- Facial, nasal, neck pain
- Eye pain, visual changes
- Anticoagulant use
- **Epistaxis**
  - Inquire about precipitating and aggravating factors and methods used to stop the bleeding—spontaneous or nose picking or other trauma; FB (foul or purulent discharge if the object has been retained for some time)—unilateral nasal discharge. Obtain head/neck HX
- SH: smoking/ETOH
- FH of bleeding disorders or leukemia
- Previous epistaxis HX
- PMH: HTN, hepatic disease, easy bruising, or prolonged bleeding after minor surgical procedures (hematologic workup)
- Meds: ASA, NSAIDs, warfarin, heparin, ticlopidine, and dipyridamole should be documented, as these not only predispose to epistaxis but make treatment more difficult

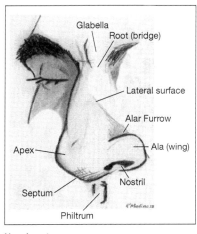

Nasal anatomy

(cont.)

NASAL PAIN/INJURY (cont.)

PE

- **General:** level of distress
- **Epistaxis:** controlling significant bleeding or hemodynamic instability should always take precedence
- **VS and SaO$_2$** (if indicated)
- **Skin:** PWD
- **HEENT:**
  - **Head:** surface trauma, TTP, bony step-off
  - **Eyes:** periorbital ecchymosis, TTP, subconjunctival hemorrhage, EOMI, diplopia, corneas grossly clear
  - **Ears:** canals, TMs clear, ruptured TM, hemotympanum, Battle's sign
  - **Nose/Face:** surface trauma, STS, ecchymosis, deformity, epistaxis, CSF leak, internal nasal injury, septal hematoma. Midface instability, movement of superior alveolar ridge. Tenderness of zygoma, maxilla, mandible
  - **Mouth/Throat:** Intraoral injury, teeth and mandible stable. Posterior pharynx clear
- **Neck:** NT, FROM. No midline point tenderness, step-off, or deformity to firm palpation of posterior cervical spine. Trachea midline. Carotids equal. No masses. No JVD. FROM of the neck without limitation or pain
- **Neuro:** A&O × 4, GCS 15, CN II–XII, grossly intact, no focal neuro deficits

MDM/DDx

Cavernous sinus thrombosis is usually a complication of an infection of the central face or paranasal sinuses. Pts at risk for this have a history of antithrombin deficiency, Factor V Leiden, protein C or S deficiency, or a genetic mutation of G202010A. Other causes include bacteremia, trauma, and infections of the ear or maxillary teeth, sinusitis, or cellulitis. **Epistaxis** is a common complaint for individuals of all ages, but in the older adult one should suspect recent anticoagulant use—especially Coumadin—or use of NSAIDs or aspirin. Older adults who have facial trauma can get posterior nasal bleeds. An isolated nasal injury is often treated as a contusion or **"clinical nasal fracture"** without radiographic confirmation. More significant injuries include **open nasal fractures** and **associated infection** or **septal hematoma,** which can lead to permanent deformity. **Nasal trauma** can also cause significant blood loss and airway management problems. **Facial fractures** associated with nasal trauma include Le Fort fractures and orbital blowout fractures with entrapment of EOMs. **Concurrent head injury** and/or **cervical spine injury** must always be considered in pts with nasal trauma.

(cont.)

NASAL PAIN/INJURY (cont.)

MANAGEMENT

- Ice, elevate HOB, analgesia. X-rays not needed for suspected nasal FX unless open FX
- **Epistaxis:** Afrin, Lidocaine Bactroban, silver nitrate/cauterization, nasal packing, or both. Poss surgery or embolization, observe rebleeding
    - Medical treatment epistaxis—pain control balanced with the concern over hypoventilation in the pt with posterior packing
    - Oral and topical antibiotics to prevent rhinosinusitis and possibly toxic shock syndrome
    - Avoidance of ASA/NSAIDs; meds to control underlying medical problems (e.g., hypertension, vitamin K deficiency)
    - Consultation with other specialists
- **Septal hematoma:** needle aspiration or I&D, Abx
- **Cavernous sinus thrombosis**
    - Abx for *Staphylococcus aureus* for gram-positive, gram-negative, and anaerobic organisms should be instituted pending the outcome of cultures. Empiric Abx therapy should include a penicillinase-resistant penicillin plus a third- or fourth-generation cephalosporin
    - If dental infection or other anaerobic infection is suspected, an anaerobic coverage should also be added. IV antibiotics minimum 3 to 4 weeks
    - Controversy on the use of anticoagulation. Locally administered thrombolytics have also been used in the treatment of CST. However, use of thrombolytics should be considered experimental and only for severe refractory cases
    - Corticosteroids after Abx coverage
    - Surgery on the cavernous sinus not helpful but I&D done

DICTATION/DOCUMENTATION

- **General:** level of distress. Awake and alert, no fever or tachycardia
- **VS and SaO$_2$** (if indicated)
- **Skin:** PWD
- **HEENT:**
    - **Head:** atraumatic, NT to palpation
    - **Eyes:** sclera and conjunctiva clear, PERRLA, EOMI without limitation or pain, no periorbital step-off, ecchymosis, or deformity. No infraorbital anesthesia
    - **Ears:** TMs normal, no hemotympanum or Battle's sign
    - **Nose/Face:** no epistaxis or CSF leak, no STS, ecchymosis, or open wounds. No bony step-off or obvious deformity. No septal hematoma. No midface instability or movement of superior alveolar ridge. No bony tenderness of zygoma, maxilla, mandible
    - **Mouth/Throat:** no intraoral trauma, teeth and mandible stable. Posterior pharynx clear
- **Neck:** FROM, NT to firm palp of bony posterior cervical spine, no paraspinal STS or TTP
- **Neuro:** A&O × 4, GCS 15, CN II–XII, grossly intact, no focal neuro deficits

(cont.)

NASAL PAIN/INJURY (cont.)

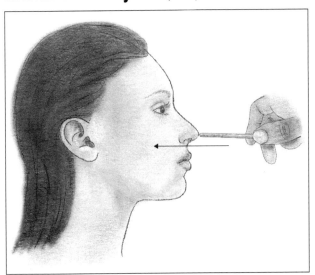

Anterior nasal packing

ANTERIOR NASAL PACKING PROCEDURE NOTE

Procedure explained and consent obtained. Local anesthetic and topical decongestant provided with Lidocaine 2% and Phenylephrine 4% (1:1 ratio) on cotton ball or atomizer. Rhino rocket, nasal tampon (Merocel), or Vaseline strip gauze inserted along floor of nare. Patient observed for 30 to 60 minutes for control of bleeding. Tolerated procedure well with no complications

◯ TIP

- If pt is advised to change anticoag dose/stop med, there should be documentation related to how this will be done (e.g., contact pt after discharge from ED to ensure that F/U care has been provided)

FACIAL PAIN

HX

- F/C, N/V
- Onset, duration, quality, location, radiation
- Provoking factors trigger points
- Severe, sharp, lancinating (stabbing), electric-shock pain
- Constant or paroxysmal
- Headache: general or focal, postauricular headache or otalgia
- Facial weakness, droop
- Change in taste or hearing
- Blurred vision, tearing, or decreased tearing
- Dental or sinus problems
- Dry mouth, burning tongue, or oral cavity
- Skin infection, HX facial HZV

PE

- **General:** level of distress
- **VS and SaO$_2$** (if indicated)
- **Skin:** PWD
- **HEENT:**
  - **Head:** scalp tenderness or trigger points
  - **Eyes:** PERRLA, tearing, redness, corneal reflex, chemosis, EOMs intact, ptosis, Bell's phenomenon (as pt closes eye, eye rolls up and in, eyelid does not close)
  - **Ears:** canals and TMs clear, pre- or postauricular lymphadenopathy
  - **Nose/Face:** nasal congestion or inflammation, frontal or maxillary sinus tenderness, STS, erythema, warmth, symmetry, facial droop, loss of nasolabial fold, facial sensation to light touch in three branches of trigeminal nerve, facial movement, trismus, TMJ, jaw click
  - **Mouth/Throat:** intraoral lesion, swelling, dental injury or infection, Wharton's duct (parotid), Stensen's duct (salivary), posterior pharynx
- **Neck:** FROM, supple, meningismus, lymphadenopathy
- **Neuro:** A&O × 4, GCS 15, CN II–XII, focal neurological deficit

(cont.)

FACIAL PAIN (cont.)

MDM/DDx

The MDM of facial pain in the older adult includes consideration of the mouth, face, and head as the origin of pain. Atypical presentation of **acute coronary syndrome** with chief complaint of face or jaw pain should not be overlooked. Nontraumatic facial pain is often caused by **oral sores, dental infection,** or **poorly fitting dentures.** Jaw pain occurs more frequently in older females. **Migraine** headaches can cause facial pain but generally decrease with advanced age. Older adults may also experience facial pain because of demyelinating disease such as **multiple sclerosis** or **tumor.** Consider **giant cell arteritis (temporal arteritis)** in older pts with new-onset headache, tenderness, or decreased pulsation in the temporal area. **Acute rhinosinusitis** or **dental infections can** result in **facial cellulitis.** Pts with any orbital involvement, such as **periorbital swelling, chemosis,** or **lateral gaze palsy (CN VI),** should be evaluated for **cavernous sinus thrombosis,** a serious complication of central face, sinus, or dental infections. **Sialadenitis** (inflammation) or **sialolithiasis** (stone) can be caused by infection or obstruction of a salivary gland. Acute onset of complete unilateral facial paralysis indicates **Bell's palsy (CV VII).** Also consider **Lyme disease** as a cause of facial paralysis. Painful facial paralysis associated with hearing loss and periauricular vesicular rash should prompt consideration of **Ramsay Hunt syndrome.** The dull ache of **TMJ dysfunction** facial pain often radiates to the ear or head and is exacerbated by chewing and eating. Any of the spectrums of **headache syndromes** can result in radiation of pain to the face

MANAGEMENT

- Refer also to "Abscess/Cellulitis," or "Dental/Intraoral Pain"
- **Sinusitis:** usually viral and requires supportive care, such as fever control, analgesia, antihistamines, decongestants, and possible intranasal steroids. Prolonged SXS may require Abx (10–14 days course): amoxicillin/clavulanate 875 BID; secondary options: clindamycin 150 to 450 mg TID (use with caution because of risk of *C. diff*); doxycycline 100 mg BID; ciprofloxacin 500 mg BID; levofloxacin 500 mg daily; ceftriaxone 1 to 2 g 12 to 24 hour; cefotaxime 2 g every 4 to 6 hours. Consider fungal etiology in immunosuppressed or DM pts. ENT referral for chronic sinusitis.
- **Bell's palsy:** protect affected eye (artificial tears, tape eye shut at night). Consider prednisone 60 mg daily × 6 days followed by tapered dose 7 to 10 days if onset of symptoms <72 hours (use with caution if immunosuppressed, DM, pregnant, infection, liver/renal disease, PUD). Possible antivirals in conjunction with corticosteroids if viral etiology suspected: acyclovir 400 mg 5×/day for 10 days or 800 mg 5×/day if HZV likely. May also use valacyclovir 500 mg BID × 5 days
- **Trigeminal neuralgia:** carbamazepine 100 mg PO BID
  - **Ramsay Hunt syndrome:** valacyclovir 1 g TID × 7 days and prednisone 1 mg/kg × 5 days
- **TMJ dysfunction:** soft diet, mouth guard, NSAIDs, muscle relaxants
- **Trigeminal neuralgia:** carbamazepine 100 mg PO BID. Topiramate 12.5 to 25 mg daily gradually increasing to 200 mg/d
- **Giant cell arteritis:** ESR (usually >50), CRP, prednisone 60 to 80 mg PO/d tapered (higher dose IV if visual changes present)

(cont.)

FACIAL PAIN (cont.)

DICTATION/DOCUMENTATION

- **General:** awake and alert, level of distress
- **VS and SaO$_2$**
- **Skin:** PWD
- **HEENT:**
  - **Head:** atraumatic, NT
  - **Eyes:** PERRLA, EOMI, no periorbital ecchymosis, step-off, deformity, subQ air
  - **Ears:** TMs clear, no hemotympanum or Battle's sign
  - **Nose: patent,** no rhinorrhea, STS, ecchymosis, abrasions or open wounds, no epistaxis or septal hematoma
  - **Face:** no swelling, bones symmetric; no flattening of malar prominences. NT to palpation and stable with attempts at manipulation. Asymmetry may be related to a new or old CVA, and decreased facial mobility may be present related to Parkinson's disease
  - **Mouth/Throat:** no intraoral trauma. Teeth and mandible are intact. No malocclusion
- **Neck:** no point tenderness, step-off or deformity to firm palpation of the cervical spine at the midline. No spasm or paraspinal muscle tenderness. FROM without limitation or pain
- **Neuro:** A&O × 4, GCS 15, CN II–XII grossly intact. Motor and sensory exam nonfocal. Reflexes are symmetric. Speech is clear and gait steady

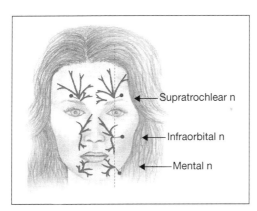

Supratrochlear n

Infraorbital n

Mental n

Locations of the facial nerves

FACIAL INJURY

HX

- Time of injury, MOI: sports, assault, MVC, fall, seizure
- HA, visual problems, neck pain, LOC
- Blood or CSF from nose or ears
- Anticoagulant use

PE

- **General:** alert, in no distress. VS stable
- **VS and SaO$_2$**
- **Skin:** PWD
- **HEENT:**
  - **Head:** scalp contusion, tenderness, open wounds, FB, bony step-off, or deformity
  - **Eyes:** VA, PERRLA, diplopia. Sclera and conjunctiva, subconjunctival hemorrhage, hyphema, EOM intact without pain or limited upward gaze. Enophthalmos or exophthalmos. Eyelid swelling, contusion, ability to open and close lids. Ability to raise eyebrows. Periorbital ecchymosis or bony step-off. Infraorbital swelling, anesthesia, palpable subcutaneous air.
  - **Ears:** canals, TMs clear, ruptured TM, hemotympanum, Battle's sign, auricular hematoma
  - **Nose:** deviation, TTP, STS, ecchymosis, open wound, epistaxis, CSF leak, septal hematoma
  - **Face:** asymmetry, STS, abrasions, ecchymosis, contusions, open wounds. Bony tenderness step-off, deformity of forehead, periorbital area, zygoma, flattened or mobile maxilla, TMJ, mandible. Midface instability, sensorimotor functions of face. Note clear drainage from mid cheek laceration in area of parotid gland.
  - **Mouth/Throat:** lip swelling or contusion. Note whether lacerations cross vermillion border or through-and-through. Tongue laceration, intraoral or dental trauma, bleeding, swelling. Patent parotid duct. Posterior pharynx clear, patent airway. Malocclusion or trismus.
- **Neck:** NT to firm midline palpation of posterior cervical spine, FROM, spasm, mass, STS
- **Chest:** CTA
- **Abd:** soft, BSA, NT
- **Back:** spinal or CVAT
- **Extremities:** FROM, NT, good strength
- **Neuro:** A&O × 4, GCS 15, CN II–XII, no focal neurological deficit

(cont.)

FACIAL INJURY (cont.)

MDM/DDx

Facial injuries range from soft tissue injury, such as **contusions** and **abrasions**, to complex **facial fractures**. Evaluation and management of an airway patency is of prime concern. Concurrent **intracranial** or **C-spine injury** should always be considered. **Eyelid injuries** involving the canthi, nasolacrimal duct, or lid margins require immediate specialty referral. Enophthalmos or exophthalmos may indicate **orbital FX.** Periorbital STS with ecchymosis, limited upward gaze, and infraorbital anesthesia are signs of **blow-out FX** with entrapment. Barotrauma can cause **rupture of the TM** on the affected side. All **nasal injuries** should be evaluated for **septal hematoma,** which can lead to permanent deformity if left untreated. Blood or CSF leaks from the nose or ears are pathognomonic for **basilar skull FX.** **Le Fort** maxillary FXs can occur as an isolated injury or in combination with other FX and are often associated with other significant injuries. **Lip injuries** are significant if laceration through-and-through or laceration involves the **vermillion border.** Most **tongue injuries** are minor and do not need sutures, especially small, central linear lacerations. Occasionally large, gaping wounds with persistent bleeding require sutures for approximation and hemostasis. **Parotid gland injury** can be caused by soft tissue injury or lacerations of the mid cheek area.

MANAGEMENT

- Airway management
- Elevate HOB, ice, analgesia
- Possible orbital/facial x-ray or CT
- Consider CSF leak
- Oral Abx if orbital FX with sinus involvement
- Anticoagulant use may require reversal depending on the medication used to decrease bleeding

DICTATION/DOCUMENTATION

- **General:** awake and alert level of distress
- **VS and SaO$_2$**
- **Skin:** PWD
- **HEENT:**
    - **Head:** atraumatic, no palpable deformities
    - **Eyes:** PERRLA, EOMI, no periorbital ecchymosis, step-off, deformity, subQ air
    - **Ears:** TMs clear, no hemotympanum or Battle's sign
    - **Nose/Face:** no STS, ecchymosis, abrasions, or open wounds. Nose NT, no swelling, no epistaxis or septal hematoma. Facial bones symmetric; no flattening of malar prominences. NT to palpation and stable with attempts at manipulation
    - **Mouth/Throat:** no intraoral trauma. Teeth and mandible are intact. No malocclusion
- **Neck:** no point tenderness, step-off, or deformity to firm palpation of the cervical spine at the midline. No spasm or paraspinal muscle tenderness. FROM without limitation or pain
- **Neuro:** A&O × 4, GCS 15, CN II–XII grossly intact. Motor and sensory exam nonfocal. Reflexes are symmetric. Speech is clear and gait steady

(cont.)

FACIAL INJURY (cont.)

▶ TIPS

- **Halo or ring sign:** blood or fluid from the nose or ear may contain CSF and indicate a basilar skull FX. Place a drop of fluid on filter or tissue paper and note clear yellowish ring of CSF layer out around blood. CSF rhinorrhea or otorrhea can be confirmed by the presence of glucose by dipstick
- **Vermillion border lip lacerations:** carefully place first suture to align lip margin to ensure optimal cosmetic outcome
- **Mandible FX:** Increased clinical suspicion for FX if pt is unable to bite and hold a tongue depressor as it is twisted

MOUTH/THROAT PAIN

HX

- Onset, duration
- Pain, swelling, temperature sensitivity, fever, difficulty swallowing, breathing, opening mouth
- Hoarseness, difficulty swallowing, muffled or "hot potato" voice, tripod position
- F/C, N/V/D
- Earache, headache, nasal discharge, congestion, sinus pain
- Dental surgery, extractions
- Tongue pain, tooth pain, mouth sores, mouth burning, dry mouth, dentures, dental implants
- Choking or coughing while eating; pocketing of food in mouth
- Sensation of lump in throat, neck pain, or swelling
- Cough, sputum production
- Rash, joint pain
- Genital discharge, oral sex
- Sick contacts
- Tobacco or alcohol use, mouth breathing, chronic allergies
- HX: esophageal problems, thyroid disease, tumor/mass, CVA, TBI, neuromuscular disorders, anemia, Sjogren's syndrome, radiation therapy
- Meds: exacerbate dry mouth such as antihistamines, chemotherapy, antianxiety

PE

- **General:** level of distress
- **VS and SaO$_2$:** fever, tachycardia, tachypnea
- **Skin:** PWD, well hydrated. No lesions or rash. No pallor or cyanosis
- **HEENT:**
  - **Head:** normocephalic without evidence of trauma
  - **Eyes:** PERRLA, sclera and conjunctiva, discharge. EOMI without limitation or pain; visual changes. No periorbital swelling. No chemosis or bloody chemosis. Proptosis, lateral gaze palsy
  - **Ears:** TMs and canals
  - **Nose:** rhinorrhea, flare
  - **Mouth/Throat:** drooling, able to handle secretions, stridor, or hoarseness. MMM or dry, intraoral lesions or ulcers. Tongue red, swollen, loss of papillae
  - **Teeth:** presence or absence of teeth or dentures; normal, broken, decayed teeth or missing teeth. Gingival swelling, erythema, bleeding, grayish pseudomembranes, foul breath. No dry or fissured or strawberry tongue, no palatal petechiae. Erythema, exudate of tonsils, and posterior pharynx. Uvula midline, no asymmetry of soft palate or postpharynx. No elevation of the floor of the mouth. Salivary ducts intact without purulence. No trismus
  - **Face:** no symmetry, tenderness, erythema, STS, warmth, loss of nasolabial fold
- **Neck:** anterior soft tissue—soft, supple, no induration or tenderness; cervical lymphadenopathy, no stiffness or meningismus, no mass or tenderness, normal thyroid
- **Chest:** CTA, wheezes/rhonchi
- **Heart:** RRR, no murmurs, rubs, or gallops
- **Abd:** soft, BSA, NT, no HSM

(cont.)

MOUTH/THROAT PAIN (cont.)

MDM/DDx

General health problems are common in older adults and are often manifested by mouth and throat problems. Many older adults have missing or weak teeth or struggle with **denture-induced stomatitis.** Dry intraoral mucosa (**xerostomia**) is not a normal part of the aging process and causes painful fissures. Burning mouth syndrome (**glossodynia**) does not involve the tongue and pain can lead to poor intake. **Glossitis** or inflammation of the tongue can be painless or painful. It is often associated with anemia, vitamin B deficiencies, malnutrition, or infection. Diminished muscle strength also makes swallowing problematic (**dysphagia**), which makes aspiration pneumonia a risk for older adults. Sore throat in older adults can be acute or chronic. Older people with complaints of sore throat are less likely to have group A beta hemolytic strep pharyngitis, and other etiologies of throat pain should also be considered. Those who are debilitated or immunosuppressed are at risk for serious or life-threatening infections of the mouth and throat. **Ludwig's angina** is a deep-space infection that often stems from a dental abscess. It extends from the floor of the mouth down to the submental area and anterior soft tissues of the neck, causing a brawny, board-like induration of soft tissues and rapid airway compromise. Although the widespread use of Hib vaccine has resulted in fewer cases of pediatric **acute epiglottitis,** the incidence in older adults remains the same because of other organisms. Inflammation of the supraglottic and laryngeal area can cause airway obstruction. **Cavernous sinus thrombosis** is a rare, septic blood clot in the deep cavity of the base of the brain; source of infection is often upper teeth, nose, or sinuses. Pts complain of headache, periorbital swelling, chemosis/bloody chemosis, decreased vision, and facial nerve palsies. **Retropharyngeal space infections** can lead to airway compromise and are associated with sore throat with normal exam, pain, stiff neck, dysphagia, hot potato voice, and stridor. Older adults can become very ill from **acute necrotizing ulcerative gingivitis** (ANUG): swollen, red gums with ulcers, foul odor, easy bleeding, and devitalized tissue. Salivary ducts can become obstructed or infected. **Sialolithiasis** is a duct stone and can affect either Wharton's duct (submandibular) or Stensen's duct (parotid); **Sialadenitis** is an inflammation or infection of a salivary duct. **Noninfectious etiologies** of sore throat include **smoking, allergies, postnasal drip, GERD,** or increased phlegm production, which can lead to **chronic irritation** of the throat. **Esophagitis, thyroiditis,** and **neoplastic** causes should be considered in older adults. Acute pharyngitis in older adults can be acute or chronic, viral or bacterial

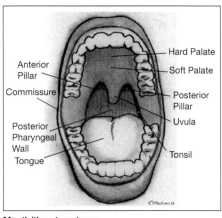

Mouth/throat anatomy

(cont.)

MOUTH/THROAT PAIN (cont.)

MANAGEMENT

▧ **Xerostomia** is difficult to treat and the underlying cause must be identified. Hydration, mucin-based artificial saliva, saliva stimulants such as ascorbic acid or gum. **Glossodynia** is also not well understood and treatment is directed to underlying causes in addition to reassurance, antidepressants, anxiolytics, and possible anticonvulsants. **Glossitis** treatment is to reduce tongue inflammation. Maintain oral hygiene; avoid irritants; use topical or oral steroids, antifungal, or Abx as indicated. Also consider underlying anemia or nutritional deficiencies. **Dysphagia:** referral for modified barium swallow and swallowing therapy

▧ **Ludwig's angina:** airway management, venous access, CBC, chemistries, coags, blood cultures if septic. Soft tissue lateral neck x-ray; CT to see extent of infection. Immunocompromised pts, which often includes older adults, should be given piperacillin/tazobactam 4.5 g IV TID or imipenem/cilastatin 500 mg IV QID (Primaxin). If concern for MRSA add vancomycin 15 to 20 mg/kg BID

▧ **Epiglottitis:** high index of suspicion for sudden deterioration and airway compromise; anticipate intubation or cricothyrotomy. Direct visualization of epiglottis by naso-pharyngoscopy/laryngoscopy soft tissue lateral neck x-ray (thumb sign or vallecula sign); possible ultz. ICU admit. Ceftriaxone 2 g IV QD; ampicillin/sulbactam 3 g QID; cefotaxime 2 g TID; add vancomycin 15 to 20 mg/kg IV if MRSA suspected

▧ **Cavernous sinus thrombosis:** treatment is based on clinical suspicion. Venous access, CBC, chemistries, blood cultures; LP and CSF analysis. MRI if poss; CT helpful to rule out other etiologies such as orbital cellulitis. Immediate Abx given empirically to cover both Gram +/− and anaerobic organisms. Nafcillin 1 to 2 g IV QID plus ceftriaxone 1 g BID. Add vancomycin 1 g BID (or use in place of Nafcillin) if concern for MRSA. Add metronidazole 500 mg IV TID to cover anaerobes related to dental infection

▧ **Retropharyngeal space infection:** airway management, venous access, CBC, chemistries, coags, blood cultures if septic. Soft tissue lateral neck x-ray: note prevertebral thickening >7 mm at C2 or >14 mm at C6; CT scan to see the extent of infection. Prepare for poss surgical drainage. If stable for outpt: Augmentin 875 mg BID or clindamycin 450 mg BID. Admitted pt: Unasyn 3 g IV QID or clindamycin 600 mg IV TID, or Pen-G 4 mu IV QID plus metronidazole 500 mg IV TID

▧ **ANUG:** PVK 500 mg QID plus metronidazole 500 mg TID × 10 days or clindamycin 450 mg TID. Add nystatin rinses QID × 1 to 2 weeks or fluconazole 200 mg QD × 1 to 2 weeks if pt is HIV+

▧ **Sialadenitis** is best treated with hydration, warm soaks, sour candy, and possible Abx

(cont.)

MOUTH/THROAT PAIN (cont.)

DICTATION/DOCUMENTATION

- **General:** level of distress; pt is awake and alert, not toxic appearing. No fever or tachycardia; no obvious respiratory distress, tripod position noted
- **VS and SaO$_2$:** note abnormal findings
- **Skin:** PWD, normal texture and turgor. No lesions or rash, no petechiae
- **HEENT:**
  - **Head:** normocephalic
  - **Eyes:** PERRLA, EOMI without limitation or complaint of pain; no lateral gaze palsy. Sclera and conjunctiva clear without injection, drainage, exudate. No proptosis. No chemosis or bloody chemosis. No periorbital STS, erythema, warmth
  - **Ears:** no pre- or postauricular lymphadenopathy, canals and TMs normal
  - **Nose/Face:** no asymmetry tenderness, erythema. No rhinorrhea, congestion
  - **Mouth/Throat:** no drooling, stridor, or hoarseness. MMM, no intra-oral lesions or ulcers. Teeth in good repair, NT to percussion
  - **Teeth:** no gingival swelling, erythema, bleeding, or foul breath. Post pharynx is clear, no erythema, exudate, or asymmetry. Uvula midline. No elevation of the floor of the mouth. Salivary ducts intact without purulence. No muffled or hot potato voice, no trismus
- **Neck:** supple, FROM, NT, no lymphadenopathy, no meningismus. Anterior soft tissues are supple, no induration tenderness. No masses, normal thyroid
- **Chest:** respirations unlabored with normal TV. No dyspnea or orthopnea. CTA without wheezes, rhonchi, rales
- **Heart:** RRR, no murmurs, rubs, or gallops
- **Abd:** BSA, NT, no HSM
- **Extremities:** moves all extremities with good strength

❍ TIPS

- Urgent ENT consultation for potential airway management problems
- Be wary of dental infections in pts with diabetes, chemotherapy with neutropenia
- Watch for airway compromise, sepsis, Ludwig's angina
- Pts taking warfarin with antibiotics need close INR monitoring. Antibiotic use can predispose older adults to *C. diff*

DON'T MISS!

Pts who take antibiotics for infection and who are taking Coumadin or warfarin need to have close monitoring of the INR before, during, and after antibiotic treatment. PCP or caregiver managing Coumadin MUST be notified about the pt's treatment in the ED and any changes made

DENTAL/INTRAORAL PAIN

DENTAL TRAUMA

- Avulsion: complete extraction of tooth, including crown and root
- Subluxation: loosened tooth
- Intrusion: tooth forced below the gingiva

FRACTURE CLASSIFICATION

- Ellis I involves only enamel. Teeth stable, nontender
- Ellis II involves enamel and dentin. Tender to touch and air. Visible exposed yellow dentin
- Ellis III involves enamel, dentin, and pulp. Tender with visible blood at center of tooth

DENTAL INFECTIONS

HX

- Pain, swelling, temperature sensitivity, fever, difficulty swallowing, breathing, opening mouth
- Ill-fitting dentures
- Dental caries
- Periodontal disease
- Dental extractions
- Dental implants
- Sjogren's syndrome
- Xerostomia

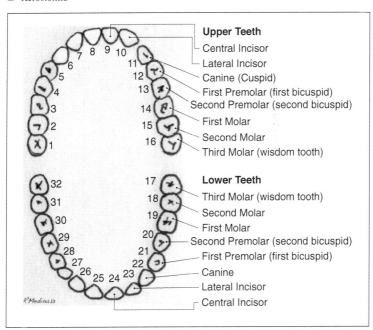

Upper Teeth
- Central Incisor
- Lateral Incisor
- Canine (Cuspid)
- First Premolar (first bicuspid)
- Second Premolar (second bicuspid)
- First Molar
- Second Molar
- Third Molar (wisdom tooth)

Lower Teeth
- Third Molar (wisdom tooth)
- Second Molar
- First Molar
- Second Premolar (second bicuspid)
- First Premolar (first bicuspid)
- Canine
- Lateral Incisor
- Central Incisor

Adult teeth chart

(cont.)

DENTAL/INTRAORAL PAIN (cont.)

PE

- **General:** use default
- **VS and SaO$_2$** (if indicated)
- **Skin:** PWD
- **Face:** swelling, neck swelling/lymphadenopathy
- **Mouth/Throat:** use default
- **Teeth:** normal, broken, or decayed teeth, gingival swelling and erythema, tender to percussion
- **Periodontal:** involves tissue surrounding the teeth
- **Periapical:** infection at root of tooth caused by caries. Often presents with facial swelling, fever, and malaise. Requires root canal or extraction. May extend to periosteum. May see small draining fistula on gingiva of periapical abscess tooth (parulis)
- **Pericoronal:** tissue over impacted tooth inflamed and infected; tooth not involved
- **Avulsed tooth:** handle tooth gently by crown; do not clean. Place in Hank's solution, milk, saline, saliva. Remove clots, replantation within 30 minutes
- **Molar infections with spread to mandibular areas sublingual:** swelling of floor of mouth, possible elevation of tongue
- **Submental:** midline induration under chin
- **Submandibular:** tenderness and swelling of angle of jaw, trismus
- **Retropharyngeal space:** sore throat with normal exam, pain, stiff neck, dysphagia, hot potato voice, stridor
- **Ludwig's angina:** brawny, board-like induration of soft tissues of anterior neck rapidly causes airway compromise
- **Upper teeth infections**
  - Facial swelling at nasolabial fold
  - May extend to infraorbital area and cause cavernous sinus thrombosis (headache, fever, periorbital swelling, chemosis/bloody chemosis, visual changes)
- **Dry socket (alveolar osteitis)**
  - Severe pain, foul odor, grayish debris at socket 4 to 5 days after extraction. Gentle cleansing, sedative dressing, such as oil of cloves, analgesia
- **Gingivitis**
  - Inflammation of tissue of gums
  - Acute necrotizing ulcerative gingivitis (ANUG): swollen, red gums with ulcers, foul odor, easy bleeding, devitalized tissue
  - **Sialolithiasis (Duct Stone):** Wharton's duct—(submandibular), Stensen's duct (parotid)
- **Sialadenitis (duct inflammation or infection)**
  - Hydration, warm soaks, massage, sour candy. Possible Abx

(cont.)

DENTAL/INTRAORAL PAIN (cont.)

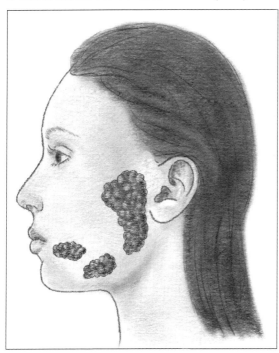

The locations of the salivary duct glands

MANAGEMENT

▣ Infection often caused by polymicrobial organisms. Abx (10-day course): PVK 500 mg PO QID; amoxicillin/clavulanate 875 PO BID; clindamycin 300 to 450 PO TID or Clindamycin 600 to 900 mg IV TID or ampicillin/sulbactam 3 g IV q6h. Abx prophylaxis indicated for Ellis II and III FXs

◉ TIPS

▣ Be wary of dental infections in pts with diabetes, or chemotherapy with neutropenia. Watch for airway compromise, sepsis, Ludwig's angina, oral infections—can lead to endocarditis

▣ Pts who take antibiotics for infection and are taking Coumadin or warfarin need to have close monitoring of the INR before, during, and after antibiotic treatment

▣ Be careful with antibiotic use, which can place pt at risk of *C. diff*

CERVICAL INJURY

HX

- Time of injury
- **MOI:** flexion, extension, rotation, lateral flexion, axial loading, penetrating trauma (type of weapon)
- **Circumstances:** sports, assault, MVC/motorcycle (speed/mph, seat belt use, location in vehicle, air-bag deployment, extent of car damage, ejection, extrication), fall, seizure, diving. Choking or hanging. Suicide/homicide
- **ALOC:** gradual or sudden, brief lucid interval
- Airway obstruction, able to speak, hoarse, dysphagia, dyspnea, HA, visual changes, face/neck pain, seizure, N/V Blood/CSF leak from nose/ears
- Back/shoulder pain (cervical, thoracic, lumbosacral). Paresthesia, weakness, paraplegia. Age >60, anticoags, drugs, ETOH. Distracting injury (e.g., extremity injury)

PE

- **General:** position of pt (e.g., full spinal precautions), level of distress, position of comfort to maintain breathing due to ankylosing spondylitis
- **VS and SaO$_2$:** bradycardia and hypotension indicate neurogenic shock; hypothermia due to poikilothermia (inability to regulate core temperature)
- **Skin:** warm, dry, flushed skin (neurogenic shock), pulse ox
- **HEENT:**
  - **Head:** scalp contusion, tenderness, open wounds, FB, bony step-off, or deformity
  - **Eyes:** PERRLA, EOMI, subconjunctival hemorrhage, petechiae, periorbital ecchymosis
  - **Ears: Battle's sign, hemotympanum, CSF leak**
  - **Nose/Face:** septal hematoma, epistaxis, CSF rhinorrhea, facial petechiae, TTP, symmetry, trauma
  - **Mouth/Throat:** drooling, stridor, intraoral bleeding; teeth and mandible
- **Neck:** surface trauma, open wounds, STS or muscle tenderness, trachea midline, tenderness over larynx; subcutaneous emphysema or crepitus. Bony TTP, step-off, or deformity to firm palpation at posterior midline. FROM without limitation or pain, flexion, extension, lateral bending, rotation, and axial load
- **Chest:** surface trauma, symmetry, tenderness, hypoventilation, lung sounds, hemoptysis
- **Heart:** RRR, no murmurs, rubs, or gallops
- **Abd:** surface trauma, BSA, tenderness, guarding, rigidity, bladder distension
- **Back:** surface trauma, spinal or CVAT
- **GU:** femoral pulses; priapism (involuntary erection—high cervical cord injury), urinary retention
- **Rectal:** saddle anesthesia, anal wink, sphincter tone, fecal incontinence
- **Extremities:** FROM, NT, distal CMS intact; assess proximal and distal muscle strength and sensation and compare to other side
- **Neuro:** A&O × 4, GCS 15, CN II–XII, no focal neuro deficits, grip strength, reflex strength or flaccid, bulbocavernosus reflex (monitor rectal sphincter tone in response to gentle tug on urinary catheter or squeeze glans penis), Babinski reflex (extension of toes)

(cont.)

CERVICAL INJURY (cont.)

MDM/DDx

Cervical spine injuries can be devastating for older adults; there is about a 25% mortality rate. Young adults often sustain cervical injuries due to high-energy forces. Older adults often have osteoporosis and can sustain injury with even low-energy force such as a fall from standing position. **Cervical pain** is often self-limiting from **muscle strain, spasm,** or **torticollis** and does not involve upper extremity paresthesia. More serious are **ligamentous injury, FX,** or **subluxation**. It is possible to have a **spinal cord injury without radiographic evidence of trauma** due to preexisting spondylotic changes in older adults. **Spinal cord injury** must be considered in every pt presenting with C/O of neck pain or significant MOI. Emergent findings are flaccid paralysis, loss of bowel and bladder reflexes and tone, and hemodynamic instability. Overlooked spine injuries can have devastating effects, and suspicion for serious injury based on mechanism of injury is essential

MANAGEMENT

- Full spinal immobilization: take care to position pt to allow breathing when there are spinal changes due to arthritis or ankylosing spondylitis
- Ice, NSAIDs
- Head CT (if indicated)
- Possible C-spine x-ray (three view or five view) based on MOI, use NEXUS criteria
- CT C-spine (standard of care)
- MRI for ligamentous injury
- NOTE: cross-table lateral film alone is not adequate

X-RAYS (C-SPINE CRITERIA)

Must be able to visualize all C1 to C7 and T1 vertebrae. C2 vertebra most commonly injured followed by C6 and C7 injury

(cont.)

CERVICAL INJURY (cont.)

DICTATION/DOCUMENTATION

- **General:** use default and state position of pt (e.g., full spinal precautions), as well as level of distress/pain. Awake and alert in no distress; no odor of ETOH
- **VS and SaO$_2$**
- **Skin:** PWD, no surface trauma
- **HEENT:**
  - **Head:** traumatic, no palpable soft tissue or bony deformities. Fontanel flat (if still open)
  - **Eyes:** PERRLA, EOMI, no subconjunctival hemorrhage, petechiae, periorbital ecchymosis
  - **Ears:** TMs clear, no hemotympanum or Battle's sign
  - **Nose/Face:** atraumatic, no asymmetry, no epistaxis or septal hematoma. Facial bones symmetric, NT to palpation and stable with attempts at manipulation
  - **Mouth/Throat:** voice clear, no pain with speaking; no drooling or stridor; no intra-oral trauma, teeth and mandible are intact
- **Neck:** no surface trauma, open wounds, soft tissue or muscle tenderness or spasm; trachea midline, no tenderness over larynx. No subQ emphysema or crepitus. No bony tenderness, step-off, or deformity to firm palpation at posterior midline. FROM without limitation or pain; normal flexion, extension, lateral bending, rotation, and axial load
- **Chest:** no surface trauma or asymmetry. NT without crepitus or deformity. Normal tidal volume. Breath sounds clear bilaterally. SaO$_2$ > 94% WNL
- **Heart:** RRR. Heart tones are normal. All peripheral pulses are intact and equal.
- **Abd:** nondistended without abrasions or ecchymosis. BSA. No tenderness, guarding, or rebound. No masses. Good femoral pulses
- **Back:** NT without step-off or deformity to firm palpation of the thoracic and lumbar spine. No contusions, ecchymosis, or abrasions are noted
- **GU:** Normal external genitalia with no blood at the meatus (if applicable). No priapism
- **Pelvis:** NT to palpation and stable to compression
- **Rectal:** normal tone. No rectal wall tenderness or mass. Stool is brown and heme negative (if applicable)
- **Extremities:** no surface trauma. FROM. Distal motor, neurovascular supply is intact
- **Neuro:** A&O × 4, GCS 15, CN II–XII grossly intact. CMS intact. No focal neuro deficits

---

C-SPINE CLEARANCE CRITERIA

Evidence-based criteria used to "clear" pt with potential cervical spine injury without radiographs; use with caution in older adults with concerning mechanism of injury or persistent pain

- No posterior midline cervical spine tenderness. No evidence of intoxication is present. Normal level of alertness
- No focal neurologic deficit is present. No painful distracting injury
- **Low risk:** simple rear-end collision, able to ambulate, gradual or delayed onset of neck pain, no specific midline cervical spine tenderness, able to rotate neck 45°
- **High risk:** >65 years; always consider associated head injury

(cont.)

CERVICAL INJURY (cont.)

DON'T MISS!

Pt must be supported to assume a position to allow breathing when there are spinal changes caused by arthritis or ankylosing spondylitis
- Flaccid, no reflexes, loss of anal sphincter tone, incontinence, priapism
- Hypotension, bradycardia, flushed, dry, and warm skin
- Ileus, urinary retention, poikilotherm
- Even a fall from a short height such as a toilet seat may result in a cervical spine injury in an older pt

Source: Adapted from Stiell, I. G., Clement, C. M., McKnight, R. D., Brison, R., Schull, M. J., Rowe, B. H., . . . Wells, G. A. (2003). The Canadian C-spine rule versus the NEXUS low-risk criteria in pts with trauma. *New England Journal of Medicine, 349*(26), 2510–2518. doi:10.1056/NEJMoa031375

COUGH/SOB

HX

- Onset, duration of cough, or SOB
- Cough dry, productive, nocturnal, hemoptysis. Sputum production—color, amount, consistency
- F/C, N/V
- Chest pain, abd pain, dizziness
- Leg pain or swelling
- Fatigue, malaise
- Dyspnea, orthopnea, PND. Postnasal drip/sinus congestion. Posttussive emesis
- Smoker, second hand smoke, environmental irritants, travel, sick contacts
- Night sweats, wt loss
- HX: hospitalizations/intubation, steroids, CPAP at night, recent surgery, home O_2 therapy
- Immunosuppressed: HIV, TB, CA, DM
- IVDA, illicit drug use
- FB aspiration/ingestion
- PE risk factors (see "Pulmonary Embolus")
- HX: GERD, recent surgery, ACE inhibitor use, DM
- FH: CA, AAA/TAD, first degree relative, HTN, connective tissue disease (e.g., Marfan's syndrome), MI/ACS, hyperlipidemia
- Risk factors
- Infectious diseases
- Altered mental status, confusion
- Falling

PE

- **General:** F/C, fatigue, malaise
- **VS and SaO$_2$**
- **Skin:** rash, cyanosis
- **HEENT:**
  - **Head:** normocephalic
  - **Eyes:** discharge, edema, erythema
  - **Ears:** TMs and canals clear
  - **Nose:** rhinorrhea, flare, boggy, hyperemic, sinuses TTP/erythema
  - **Mouth/Throat:** MMM, erythema, exudate, stridor
- **Neck:** supple, FROM, lymphadenopathy, meningismus, JVD
- **Chest:** retractions, accessory muscle use, TV, grunting, lung sounds clear, wheezes, rales, rhonchi, pleural friction rub, dyspnea, orthopnea, tripod. Able to speak easily in full sentences
- **Heart:** RRR, no murmurs, rubs, or gallops
- **Abd:** soft, NT
- **Extremities:** STS, edema, status of upper extremity circulation

(cont.)

COUGH/SOB (cont.)

MDM/DDx

SOB is not part of the normal aging process. Older adults with SOB require prompt evaluation for **pneumonia, pulmonary emboli, CHF, COPD exacerbation, ACS,** and **anemia** of chronic disease. Aspiration pneumonia is seen in older pts and foreign-body aspiration in pts with **dementia** (e.g., food bolus, dentures). Other potential Dxs for cough and SOB range from benign and self-limiting problems such as upper respiratory infection (URI) or mild asthma to resp **failure.** Sudden, severe chest pain/SOB with pain radiating to the abd/back may indicate AAA/TAD

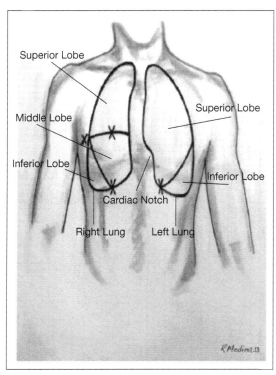

The lobes of the lungs

(cont.)

COUGH/SOB (cont.)

MANAGEMENT

- **ABCs, stat EKG** if indicated
- **URI:** supportive care, fever control, antihistamine if allergic
- **Asthma/COPD:** bronchodilators, steroids, Abx for PNA, CXR if F/C or suspect infiltrate
    - Admit if refractory to HHN, retraction, hypoxia, fatigue, repeat recent visits, HX resp failure
- **Bronchitis:** supportive care, fever control, cough suppression. Bronchodilators, steroids, NSAIDs, mucolytics
    - Add Abx if AECB, DM, CHF, steroids, >65 years with acute cough, Abx (7–10 days): azithromycin 500 mg × 1 then 250 mg QD × 4 days; amoxicillin 875 mg BID; TMP/SMX (DS) 1 to 2 tab; amoxicillin/clavulanate 875 mg BID; levofloxacin 500 mg QD. CXR if F/C, CP, suspect infiltrate
- **Pertussis:** if cough >2 weeks: azithromycin 500 mg × 1 then 250 mg QD × 4 days (<6 months 10 mg/kg × 5 days); erythromycin 500 mg QID (>1 month 10 mg/kg) × 14 days; TMP/SMX (DS) 1 to 2 tabs BID × 14 days
- **CAP:** based on severity and need for hospitalization: hypoxia, vomiting, septic, >65 years, unreliable
    - **"Sick CAP pts":** O_2, IV NS bolus, CBC, BMP, lactate, blood/sputum cx, CXR
    - **Outpt CAP:** Abx choice based on many factors, such as outpt or inpt treatment, age, CAP, AIDS, aspiration, lung disease, recent admit. Abx (7–10 days): azithromycin 500 mg PO × 1 then 250 mg PO daily × 4 days, doxycycline 100 mg PO BID, levofloxacin 500 mg PO daily, amoxicillin 500 mg PO TID, amoxicillin/clavulanate 875 mg PO BID. CXR: document baseline; may defer if stable and treatment unchanged. Consider resistance to macrolides
- Follow evidence-based protocols for treatment of infections and early consultation
- **AAA/TAD:** CXR, ultz, CT, angiogram, MRA

ADULT COMMUNITY-ACQUIRED PNEUMONIA
RISK FACTORS

- Male > female, nursing home
- HX: cancer, CVA, CHF, liver or renal Dx
- ALOC; hypo/hyperthermia, heart rate (HR) >124, respiratory rate (RR) >30, blood pressure (B/P) <90; SaO_2 <90, pH <7.35; BUN >30; Na <130; Glucose >250; Hct <30; pleural effusion

(cont.)

COUGH/SOB (cont.)

DICTATION/DOCUMENTATION

- **General:** awake and alert, in no obvious resp distress
- **VS and SaO$_2$**
- **Skin:** PWD, no cyanosis or pallor
- **HEENT:**
    - **Head:** normocephalic
    - **Eyes:** PERRLA, sclera and conjunctiva clear
    - **Ears:** canals and TMs normal
    - **Nose:** no rhinorrhea or nasal flare
    - **Mouth/Throat:** MMM, posterior pharynx clear
- **Neck:** supple, FROM, no JVD, trachea midline
- **Chest:** no orthopnea or dyspnea. Able to speak in complete sentences, no retractions or accessory muscle use, no tripod position, no grunting or stridor. CTA bilaterally, no wheezes, rhonchi, rales
- **Heart:** RRR
- **Abdomen:** soft, NT
- **Extremities:** no swelling, edema, tenderness

CXR INTERPRETATION NOTE

Note whether one- or two-view chest film done:

No bony abnormality (i.e., no DJD, lytic lesions, rib FX). Heart is normal size, no cardiomegaly

Lungs reveal no pneumothorax, hyperinflation, infiltrate, effusion, mass, or cavitation (TB) or FB aspiration. Mediastinum not widened, no pneumomediastinum, no hilar adenopathy or tracheal deviation

DON'T MISS!

- Acute coronary syndrome
- Congestive heart failure
- Pulmonary embolus
- Pneumothorax
- FB (dentures)/aspiration

CHEST PAIN

HX

- P = **Provoking/precipitating factors;** alleviating factors
- Q = **Quality**—heavy, achy tight (esp in women)
- R = **Radiation/region**—migration or movement of pain (AAA/TAD)
- S = **Severity**—pain scale 1 to 10
- T = **Timing:** of onset, duration, time of day
- Jaw pain, hoarseness, painful swallowing, heartburn, hematemesis, melena SOB, exertional dyspnea = risk factor, F/C, N/V, indigestion, diaphoresis, dizzy, syncope, cough, hemoptysis. Back/flank pain, abd/epigastric pain, fatigue, malaise, exertional dyspnea, PND, leg pain/STS
- Recent viral illness or surgical procedures; prosthetic heart valve, pacemaker, implantable defibrillator LVAD
- FH: AAA/TAD, first-degree relative, prior AAA/TAD, connective tissue disease (e.g., Marfan's syndrome), early sudden death
- SH: smoker, ETOH, IVDA, or illicit drug use
- HX: ACS/MI, CAD, HTN, PE, obesity, postmenopausal, previous EKG, cardiac workup, caths

PE

- **General:** position of pt, level of distress
- **VS and SaO$_2$:** BP both arms
- **Skin:** pale, cool, diaphoretic, cyanosis
- **HEENT:**
  - **Head:** normocephalic
  - **Eyes:** pupils PERRLA and EOMI
  - **Ears:** TMs and canals clear
  - **Nose:** patent
  - **Mouth/Throat:** MMM
- **Neck:** FROM, trachea midline, bruits, JVD, subcutaneous emphysema
- **Chest:** NT, retractions, accessory muscle use, TV, CTA, wheezes, rales, rhonchi, pleural friction rub. Dyspnea, orthopnea
- **Heart:** RRR, no murmurs, rubs, or gallops
- **Abdomen:** SNT, epigastric mass, pulsation; stool OB
- **Extremities:** STS, edema, status of upper extremity circulation, femoral pulses
- **Neuro:** no LOC and no focal neuro deficits

(cont.)

CHEST PAIN (cont.)

MDM/DDx

Chest pain in older people is more often caused by serious problems. The incidence and severity of CAD increases with age. Older adults must be evaluated quickly to identify emergent causes of chest pain that can lead **to sudden death.** STEMI/ACS should be considered in pts with left or mid chest pressure, SOB, and diaphoresis. Sudden, severe chest pain radiating to the back may indicate **AAA/TAD.** PE can present with a wide range of SXS and may be very subtle; it should be included in every evaluation of chest pain/SOB. A high index of suspicion for PE must be had for older adults with a history of CHF, malignancy, obesity, pacemaker, or hyperviscosity due to multiple myeloma. **Spontaneous pneumothorax** is more common in younger adults who are thin, smokers, or have Marfan's syndrome. Pts with **acute cardiac tamponade** may present classic findings of dyspnea, distended neck veins, and signs of shock. **Esophageal rupture,** an uncommon cause, may be indicated by lower chest/upper abd pain, vomiting, trouble swallowing or hoarseness, crepitus, and signs of shock. More common and less serious etiologies include **pneumonia, GERD, cholecystitis,** and **musculoskeletal pain** or **trauma.** Low-grade fever with pleuritic mid chest pain that is worse with inspiration and relieved by leaning forward may indicate **pericarditis.** Chest pain with low-grade fever may also indicate **endocarditis.** Sudden SOB, altered mental status, or heart murmur in these pts should prompt a search for petechiae, splinter hemorrhages, Osler nodes, Janeway lesions, or splenomegaly. **Cocaine-related ischemia** is more common in younger people who may present with either tachycardia or bradycardia and who are often hypertensive

MANAGEMENT

- Geriatric pts may have vague symptoms related to an acute MI. Some of these symptoms include fatigue, nausea, and a decrease in functional status. The pt may complain more often of shortness of breath than chest pain
- Stat EKG within 10 minutes of arrival—identify STEMI (activate STEMI team, consult/transfer)
- O$_2$, IV, EKG monitor, SaO$_2$ ASA (hold if dissection)
- Nitroglycerin (NTG; hold NTG if hypotensive, inferior MI, erectile dysfunction meds), CBC, BMP, cardiac enzymes, troponin (not present in serum for 3 hours; peaks 12 hours), coags, consider BNP, D-dimer, T&C portable two-view CXR, serial EKGs, old EKGs if available (but do not delay treatment)
- Possible CT, ult. Other: analgesia, vasopressors, anticoagulants. Cooling measures postarrest

EKG INTERPRETATION NOTE

Normal rate, normal rhythm, normal axis, and normal intervals. There was no significant ST segment or T wave changes to suggest acute ischemia or infarction

CXR INTERPRETATION NOTE

One- or two-view chest film done
    No bony abnormality (i.e., no DJD, lytic lesions, rib FX), heart is normal size, no cardiomegaly
    Lungs reveal no pneumothorax, hyperinflation, infiltrate, effusion, mass, or cavitation or FB aspiration. Mediastinum not widened, no pneumomediastinum, no hilar adenopathy or tracheal deviation

(cont.)

CHEST PAIN (cont.)

DICTATION/DOCUMENTATION

- **General:** awake and alert, in no obvious distress
- **VS and SaO$_2$:** B/P both arms
- **Skin:** PWD, no diaphoresis, cyanosis, or pallor
- **HEENT:**
  - **Head:** normocephalic
  - **Eyes:** PERRLA, sclera, and conjunctiva clear
  - **Ears:** canals and TMs normal
  - **Nose:** patent
  - **Mouth/Throat:** MMM, posterior pharynx clear
- **Neck:** supple, FROM, no JVD, trachea midline, no bruits
- **Chest:** no orthopnea or dyspnea noted; no retractions or accessory muscle use. NT, no crepitus. CTA bilaterally, no wheezes, rhonchi, rales
- **Heart:** RRR, no murmurs, rubs, or gallops
- **Abd:** soft, BSA, NT, no epigastric tenderness, mass, pulsation; femoral pulses
- **Back:** no CVAT
- **Extrems:** no swelling, edema, tenderness
- **Neuro:** no LOC and no focal neuro deficits

HEART Score (calculate for patients >21 years old with complaint of chest pain to stratify risk of ACS)

H: Concerning or suspicious history
E: EKG: no ST deviation but LBBB, LVH, repolarization changes (e.g., digoxin), or ST deviation present not due to LBBB, LVH, or digoxin
A: Age < 45 or >65 years old
R: Risk factors such as HTN, DM, hypercholesterolemia, obesity, smoking, family history, PMH of MI, CABG, CVA/TIA, PAD
T: Troponin level

See www.mdcalc.com/heart-score-major-cardiac-events

DON'T MISS!

- Stat EKG within 10 minutes
- Identify STEMI
- If STEMI—cath lab within 90 minutes
- Obtain old EKG for comparison

PULMONARY EMBOLUS

HX

A thorough history regarding PE risk factors is essential because many pts have vague or atypical physical complaints ranging from fever and cough to seizures or altered mental status, as well as cardiovascular collapse.

- Age >60 years
- Recent surgery or trauma, CVA within last month
- HX: DVT/PE, prior history, syncope, AMI, valve dysfunction, CHF, COPD, SLE, ulcerative colitis, or IBD
- Hypercoagulopathy, varicose veins
- Active cancer, chemotherapy, radiation therapy
- Recent prolonged bed rest, immobilization, cross-country travel, pregnancy, postpartum within 1 month, estrogen therapy, obesity, smoking, IVDA
- Valve dysfunction, heart disease, AFib, heart failure cough, F/C, SOB, recent
- Infection

PE

- **General:** level of distress, anxiety
- **VS and SaO$_2$:** fever, tachypnea, tachycardia
- **Skin:** PWD or pale, cool, moist
- **HEENT:**
  - **Head:** normocephalic
  - **Eyes:** pupils PERRLA and EOMI
  - **Ears:** TMs and canals clear
  - **Nose:** patent
  - **Mouth/Throat:** MMM
- **Neck:** supple, no lymphadenopathy, no meningismus, no JVD
- **Chest:** tachypnea, nonproductive cough, wheezes or rales, hypoxia, hemoptysis. Sharp, pleuritic chest pain
- **Heart:** tachycardia
- **Abd:** pain
- **Back:** flank pain
- **Extremities:** STS, edema; unilateral/bilateral, TTP calf/medial thigh, Homan's sign (pain with forced dorsiflexion of foot) unreliable. Possible overlying warmth, erythema, discoloration or blanched appearance; possible superficial thrombophlebitis with palpable, tender cords
- **Neuro:** syncope, seizures, altered mental status

(cont.)

PULMONARY EMBOLUS (cont.)

MDM/DDx

The diagnosis of PE in older adults is clinically challenging because presenting signs and symptoms are variable and often vague and nonspecific. PE risk factors in the aged include obesity, smoking, immobilization, and history of PE or DVT, malignancy, hyperviscosity caused by multiple myeloma, CHF, and nephrotic syndrome; although not all pts have known risk factors, recent travel, trauma, and surgical procedures should be considered. Many older adult pts with PE do not have the "classic" findings of sudden **pleuritic chest pain, dyspnea, and hypoxia**. As a result, this common and potentially fatal problem is often overlooked. Relevant history of risk factors for PE is the foundation for the diagnosis. **Recurrent PE** should always be considered in pts with a history of previous PE. The diagnosis of PE should be considered a diagnosis of exclusion when other causes have been confirmed. Problems causing similar signs and symptoms include **musculoskeletal chest pain, pleurisy, pericarditis, pneumonia, hyperventilation**, and others

MANAGEMENT

With a careful history and assessment, some low risk patients may not require any diagnostic testing. If any concern for possible PE, use the Wells' criteria and PERC rules for risk stratification

WELLS' CRITERIA RISK LEVELS

- **Low risk:** PERC negative—stop workup. Note: PERC criteria applies to adults <50 years of age
- **Moderate risk, comorbidities:** D-dimer (use age-adjusted cutoff to indicate need for imaging)
- **High risk:** CXR, CT angio (ventilation/perfusion [V/Q] scan only if CT not available or contraindication to contrast dye), pulmonary angiography; CBC, chem panel, ABG, troponin, BNP, EKG, possible ultz for DVT. Immediate therapeutic anticoagulation with heparin or LMWH; thrombolytics; possible surgical intervention

---

PULMONARY EMBOLISM RULE-OUT CRITERIA (PERC)

If all criteria met in low-risk pt = <2% risk for PE = no PE workup
- Age <50 years
- Heart rate (HR) <100 BPM
- SaO_2 >94%
- No prior PE or DVT
- No SXS DVT
- No hemoptysis
- No recent trauma/surgery
- No hormone use

Source: Adapted from Wells, P. S., Anderson, D. R., Rodger, M., Stiell, I., Dreyer, J. F., Barnes, D., . . . Kovacs, M. J. (2001). Excluding pulmonary embolism at the bedside without diagnostic imaging: Management of patients with suspected pulmonary embolism presenting to the emergency department by using a simple clinical model and D-dimer. *Annals of Internal Medicine, 135*(2), 98–107. doi:10.7326/0003-4819-135-2-200107170-00010; Wolf, S. J., McCubbin, T. R., Feldhaus, K. M., Faragher, J. P., & Adcock, D. M. (2004). Prospective validation of Wells criteria in the evaluation of patients with suspected pulmonary embolism. *Annals of Emergency Medicine, 44*(5), 503–510. doi:10.1016/j.annemergmed.2004.04.002

(cont.)

PULMONARY EMBOLUS (cont.)

DICTATION/DOCUMENTATION

- **General:** awake and alert, level of distress, anxiety
- **VS and SaO$_2$:** awake, alert; elevated temp, tachypnea, tachycardia
- **Skin:** PWD. No diaphoresis, cyanosis, or pallor
- **HEENT:**
  - **Head:** normocephalic
  - **Eyes:** pupils PERRLA and EOMI
  - **Ears:** TMs and canals clear
  - **Nose:** patent
  - **Mouth/Throat:** MMM
- **Neck:** no JVD
- **Chest:** resps unlabored, normal TV. Pt able to speak easily in complete sentences; no orthopnea or dyspnea. Lungs are clear bilaterally, no wheezing or rales. No cough or hemoptysis. No hypoxemia
- **Heart:** RRR, no murmurs, rubs, or gallops.
- **Abd:** flat, BSA, NT
- **Back:** no spinal or flank pain, no CVAT
- **Extrems:** no STS, edema, or evidence of thrombophlebitis
- **Neuro:** A&O × 4, GCS 15, no focal neuro deficits, no seizure

DON'T MISS!

- PE that masquerades as pneumonia
- PE that presents as syncope

ABDOMINAL PAIN/INJURY

HX

MEDICAL

- Onset: sudden or gradual
- Duration: hours to days is more urgent, exacerbation of chronic problems. Localized or diffuse pain
- Characteristics: intermittent, sharp, dull, achy. Referred pain to groin/scrotum, right or left scapula. GI: N/V, emesis: bloody, undigested food, bilious, projectile vomiting
- Constipation/diarrhea, bloody diarrhea, bowel changes, bloating, passing gas, refusing/decreasing food/fluids, removing food from the mouth
- Flank pain, urinary urgency, frequency, burning pain, hematuria, testicular pain, pain begins abruptly then resolves or migrates to abd/back = TAD. Recent use of NSAIDs, cough, chest pain, or pressure
- Sexual HX, vaginal bleeding/discharge, unprotected sexual intercourse
- HX of same pain with new progression
- ETOH, tobacco, drugs, FH, meds
- **PMH:** AFib, DM, CA, Hep C, GB, pancreatitis, obesity
  - AAA, TAD, first-degree relative, prior
  - HTN, connective tissue disease (e.g., Marfan's syndrome)
- PSH—abd surgeries
- Time of last food and fluid intake
- Recent travel
- **Trauma:**
- MOI (blunt vs. penetrating)
- Blunt: assault, maltreatment, fall, auto/ped, MVC. Penetrating: stabbing, GSW, missile inj

(cont.)

ABDOMINAL PAIN/INJURY (cont.)

PE

- **General:** alert, writhing, still, confused, combative
- **VS and SaO$_2$:** fever, tachycardia, hypotension, pulse ox, BP both arms if suspect thoracic aortic aneurysm
- **Skin:** PWD or pale, cool, moist; jaundice, dehydration
- **HEENT:**
  - **Head:** normocephalic
  - **Eyes:** pupils PERRLA and EOMI
  - **Ears:** TMs and canals clear
  - **Nose:** patent
  - **Mouth/Throat:** MMM
- **Neck:** supple, no lymphadenopathy, no meningismus, no JVD
- **Chest:** CTA bilaterally, no rales, rhonchi, or wheezing
- **Heart:** RRR, no murmurs, rubs, or gallops.
- **Abd:**
  - **Medical:** soft/flat/distended; BS, guarding, rebound, rigid, tender, pulsatile masses, scars, surface trauma, hernia
  - **Trauma:** PE findings may be unreliable because of MOI. Note associated injuries, distracting pain, AMS, ETOH. Note surface trauma distention, tenderness to palpation; guarding, rebound, rigidity. Spleen—L referred shoulder pain (Kehr's sign). Periumbilical ecchymosis (Cullen's sign). Flank ecchymosis (Grey Turner's sign)
- **Extremities:** upper extremities circulation

Localized Pain

- **RUQ:** GB, FHCS, hepatitis, PNA, pyelonephritis, renal calc
- **LUQ:** spleen, gastritis, PUD, PNA, pyelonephritis, renal calc, heart failure, liver congestion
- **RLQ:** appy, renal calc, inguinal hernia, GYN (PID, cyst, torsion, TOA), test torsion
- **LLQ:** diverticulitis, AAA, inguinal hernia, renal calc, GYN (menses, PID, cyst, ectopic, torsion, TOA), test torsion, Crohn's disease, colitis
- **Epigastric:** GERD, PUD, gastritis, pancreatitis, MI/ACS
- **Periumbilical:** pancreatitis, SBO, appy, AGE, AAA, perforated viscous, nonspecific
- **Umbilical pain:** poss appy (tip of appendix may be behind umbilicus)
- **Suprapubic:** UTI, retention, prostatitis, PID (longer duration of SXS, CMT, and adnexal tenderness), uterine problems
- **Chest/Back/Flank:** AAA: aorta WNL if L of midline but abnormal if palp R of midline or >3 cm

DIFFUSE PAIN

- AGE, DKA, BO, IBS, ischemia, SCD, perforated viscus, Murphy's sign, tenderness at McBurney's point
- **GU:** normal external genitalia, urinary meatus, femoral pulses, no hernia, normal testicles, cremasteric reflex
- **Rectal:** blood, pain, or mass (fecal impaction, tumor, prostate, pelvic abscess)
- **Vaginal:** CMT, os closed, no adnexal fullness or TTP
- **Back:** CVAT, ecchymosis

(cont.)

ABDOMINAL PAIN/INJURY (cont.)

MDM/DDx

Abdominal pain is a challenging complaint in pts of any age; the increasingly aging population makes this an even more common occurrence. Older adults are more likely to have significant comorbidities and impaired immune systems. Some older adults delay seeking medical attention, report nonspecific complaints, experience minimal pain, or have AMS. Early identification of pts with potentially life-threatening causes of abd pain is the priority. Hemodynamic stability and lack of serious comorbidities are reassuring findings. **Biliary tract disease** is still one of the most common etiologies for abd pain in older adults as pts may have **gallstones.** Older pts may present with vague pain and require a high index of suspicion for this diagnosis. Colicky abd pain may also be due to **renal calculi.** Melena should prompt evaluation for **PUD;** older adults often have minimal or no abd pain even with perforation. **Diverticular disease** is also common and affects over half of all older adults. Compared to younger pts with diverticulitis, older adults are less likely to have fever, elevated WBCs, or blood in stool. **Mesenteric ischemia** is a rare but catastrophic cause of acute abd in older adults; AFib is a risk factor. ABO, such as sigmoid volvulus, can lead to **bowel perforation** if not detected. It is important to consider other GU/GYN etiologies, such as **hernia or ovarian torsion,** in pts with a complaint of right lower abd pain. Metabolic problems like **DKA** can present with vague, diffuse abd pain, and vomiting. Intractable vomiting: **cannabinoid hyperemesis syndrome.** Diagnosis of serious surgical problems, such as appendicitis, strangulated hernia, or testicular torsion, is vital. **Appendicitis** is less common in older pts but is associated with much higher mortality. Intractable pain, uncontrolled vomiting, unstable vital signs, or AMS in older adults are indications for hospital admission. Consideration of extra-abd etiologies, such as pulmonary SXS with tachypnea and hypoxia, should prompt the investigation of **PE** or **pneumonia. AMI/ACS** may present with upper abd pain. Sudden severe chest pain radiating to the back may indicate **AAA/TAD**

MANAGEMENT

- **Low risk:** analgesia, antiemetics, UA, FBSG
  - Consider age, pain severity, hemodynamic stability, risk for serious etiology
- **High risk:** NPO, IV NS, analgesia, antiemetic, CBC, BMP, LFT/lipase, lactate. Dip UA/UCG, FSBS
  - Recheck abd, pain, fluid tolerance, poss GC/chlamydia; CXR: infiltrate, free air, KUB/Abd, EKG, RUQ ultz; CT abd/pelvis
  - AAA: CXR, CT, angiogram, MRA. Surgical consult; Abx for sepsis
- **Trauma:** ABCs
  - O_2, IVs, EKG, monitor, gastric tube (as indicated), urinary catheter. Labs: blood type and screen, CBC, chem panel, lactate level. UA.
  - Imaging: CXR, FAST ultz exam (CT if stable)
  - Peritoneal lavage (as indicated)
  - Surgical consult for possible exploratory laparotomy (as indicated)

(cont.)

ABDOMINAL PAIN/INJURY (cont.)

DICTATION/DOCUMENTATION

- **General:** appearance, behavior, level of distress, anxiety, agitated. LOC and in no acute distress
- **Nontoxic appearing**
- **VS and SaO$_2$:** VSS or elevated temp, tachypnea, tachycardia. Compare B/P bilaterally in extrems
- **Skin:** PWD, no diaphoresis, cyanosis, or pallor, no skin lesions/rashes
- **HEENT:**
  - **Head:** atraumatic, NT
  - **Eyes:** sclera and conjunctiva clear, corneas grossly clear. PERRLA, EOMIs, no nystagmus or ptosis
  - **Ears:** canals and TMs normal. No hemotympanum or Battle's sign
  - **Nose/Face:** atraumatic, NT, no asymmetry
  - **Mouth/Throat:** MMM, posterior pharynx clear, normal gag reflex, no intraoral trauma
- **Neck:** supple, FROM, NT, no lymphadenopathy, no meningismus
- **Chest:** CTA, no wheezes, rhonchi, rales. Normal TV, no retractions or accessory muscle use. No respiratory depression
- **Heart:** RRR, no murmurs, rubs, or gallops
- **Abd:** soft, flat, without distension, ascites. No surface trauma, scars, incisions. BSA and present in all four quadrants. No tenderness, guarding, rigidity to palpation. No pulsatile masses noted. No hepatosplenomegaly. Negative Murphy's sign. No periumbilical tenderness. No rebound TTP. No tenderness over McBurney's point. No suprapubic TTP
- **GU:** Good femoral pulses bilaterally. No hernia noted
- **Back:** no spinal or CVAT
- **Extremities:** FROM with good strength, distal motor neurovascular supply intact
- **Neuro:** A&O × 4, GCS 15, CN II–XII grossly intact. No focal neuro deficits. Normal muscle strength and tone. Normal DTRs, negative Babinski, normal finger-to-nose coordination or heel-to-shin glide. Speech, gait, Romberg neg, no pronator drift

ABDOMINAL X-RAY INTERPRETATION NOTE

If abd plain film ordered—document condition of aorta (e.g., calcification)

❯ TIPS

- Be wary of abd pain in older adults who do not appear febrile (confirm via rectal temperature)
- Older adults may not have classic signs of an acute abd (e.g., severe pain)
- Hemodynamic instability and severe abd pain = emergent pt (immediate surgical consult)
- Life-threatening: abd trauma. AAA/TAD, mesenteric ischemia, perforated peptic ulcer, pancreatitis
- Negative ultz/CT does not eliminate Dx of appy
- Constipation and AGE are diagnoses of exclusion in older adults
- Review meds for any changes that may cause abd pain or interfere with PO intake
- Recent HX of Abx use; consider *Clostridium diff*
- Timing of diarrhea: after eating, nighttime diarrhea may be infectious

(cont.)

ABDOMINAL PAIN/INJURY (cont.)

DON'T MISS!

- Appendicitis
- Gallbladder disease
- Bowel perforation
- Mesenteric ischemia
- TAD/classic triad of AAA (pain, hypotension, pulsatile abd mass)

GENITOURINARY PROBLEMS

HX

- **Onset:** sudden or gradual pain
- **Duration:** hours to days = more urgent, exacerbation/recurrence of chronic prob
- **Localized or diffuse: unilateral or bilateral**
- Abd, flank/back, penile/scrotal, urinary meatus. Referred pain to abd/back/groin/scrotum
- **Characteristics:** severity, pattern, and location of pain
- Timing: intermittent, sharp, dull, achy, pain with urination or intercourse
- Aggravating or relieving factors
- F/C, N/V, fatigue, myalgias, malaise
- Urinary urgency, frequency, dysuria, hematuria, clots, urinary retention
- Appetite, fluid intake, urinary output
- Use of adult diapers, external or indwelling catheter
- Constipation/diarrhea, bowel changes, blood, pus
- Recent illness, instrumentation, surgery
- Vaginal or penile bleeding or discharge
- Testicular pain, swelling, redness; feeling of heaviness or mass in scrotum, perineal or rectal pain. HX sexual partners, HIV
- HX uterine/rectal prolapse, paraphimosis
- Trauma: penetrating, blunt trauma, straddle injury. Do not confuse mild trauma with torsion.
- FH: AAA/TAD first-degree relative, prior AAA/TAD, HTN

PE

- **General:** alert, writhing, still, lethargic, confusion, combative, wandering
- **VS and SaO$_2$:** fever, signs of shock
- **Skin:** PWD or pale, cool, moist; jaundice, dehydration
- **Chest:** lung sounds
- **Abd:** surface trauma, scars, flat or distended; bowel sounds; guarding, rebound, rigid, tenderness, mass, organomegaly
- **GU:** femoral pulses, lymphadenopathy, lesions/rash, inguinal canal hernia, external genitalia, perineum, urinary meatus, skin breakdown, bullae, crepitus, surface trauma, erythema, warmth
- **Male:** circumcised/uncircumcised, foreskin retraction, penis, urinary meatus, discharge, phimosis/paraphimosis. Scrotum/testes: swelling of testis and/or scrotum; high-riding or horizontal lie of testicle. Small, tender palp mass at upper pole. Palp "bag of worms" (varicocele). Effect of elevation of testis on pain level. Scrotal abscess/mass/Fournier gangrene. Transillumination (hydrocele). Soft, boggy prostate, cremasteric reflex: normal elevation of testis when inner thigh stroked
- **Female:** CMT, bleeding, no adnexal fullness or TTP, prolapsed bladder or rectum
- **Back:** spinal or CVAT
- **Rectal:** blood, pain, mass (fecal impaction, tumor, enlarged prostate, pelvic abscess)

(cont.)

GENITOURINARY PROBLEMS (cont.)

MDM/DDx

Age-related changes in the genitourinary system of older adults places them at risk for functional or structural problems, infection, incontinence, prostate enlargement, and malignancy. Priority should be given to early identification of pts with emergent causes of genitourinary pain. Sudden, severe chest pain radiating to the back/flank may indicate **AAA/TAD. UTIs** are one of the most common admission diagnoses in older adults; confusion or altered mental status is a common finding. After age 60 years, men experience as many infections as women. **Complicated UTIs** include recurrent or failed treatment, multiple urinary tract infections, UTI treatment that has required the use of IV antibiotics to manage, indwelling urinary catheter, elevated BUN/creatinine, and urinary retention. Ascending urinary tract infection (**pyelonephritis**) is a serious disease characterized by F/C, N/V, flank pain, or CVAT, N/V, and signs of sepsis. Acute pyelonephritis is a serious problem in older adults, especially men, because the condition is often complicated by BPH and urethral obstruction or urinary retention. **Prostatitis** may be caused by UTI, urinary catheter, recent prostate biopsy, or surgery; most common cause is *E. coli*. **Acute urinary retention** is a medical emergency; risk is highest after age 70 years and can be caused by infection or prostatic hypertrophy, medications such as antihistamines, decongestants, or tricyclics. Urinary retention is rare in females and raises concern for serious neurologic impairment such as spinal cord compression. Local redness and swelling of the glans penis indicates **balanitis**; it is called **balanoposthitis** when the foreskin is also infected. This local infection may lead to **phimosis,** an inability to retract the foreskin. A urological emergency in uncircumcised males is **paraphimosis,** the inability to return a retracted foreskin over the head of the penis. This is often an iatrogenic problem but also occurs after sexual activity and in nursing home pts. **Penile trauma** ranges from **urethral FBs to constrictive devices that may be used in an attempt to control incontinence.** Catastrophic causes for scrotal or testicular pain in older men include AAA and Fournier gangrene. Maintain a high index of suspicion for **AAA** in older adults who have sudden groin pain associated with altered mental status and signs of shock. **Fournier gangrene may occur** in any older or immunosuppressed pt who appears toxic with scrotal or perineal soft tissue blisters or necrosis. Older men more commonly experience testicular or scrotal pain from infection or trauma or structural problems. **Epididymitis** and/or **orchitis and prostatitis** in older adults can be noninfectious because of urine reflux into ejaculatory ducts. If sexually active, consider sexually transmitted diseases, such as gonorrhea or chlamydia, which may be associated with systemic signs/SXS (e.g., pain, F/C). Extra testicular etiologies for referred pain include **ureteral colic** and **appendicitis. Consider incarcerated inguinal hernia** if there is sudden, severe pain, N/V, and a nonreducible mass in the inguinal area or scrotum. **Testicular tumors** may cause painless or painful scrotal swelling. All pts with scrotal pain must be evaluated for **testicular torsion**, which is a surgical emergency but uncommon in older adult males and may have atypical or subtle presentation. Classic findings are sudden onset of unilateral testicular pain with a high-riding or horizontally displaced testis

(cont.)

GENITOURINARY PROBLEMS (cont.)

MANAGEMENT

- ▓ **Signs of urosepsis:** ABCs, fluid resuscitation, baseline labs with cultures
- ▓ **Urinary retention:** relieve immediately, degree and duration of retention leads to renal dysfunction. Urinary catheterization, irrigate as needed. Consider calculi, UTI, urosepsis
- ▓ **UTI:** outpt if tolerate fluids and not toxic. TMP/SMX (DS) 1 tab PO BID × 3 days; nitrofurantoin 100 mg PO BID × 7 days. Amoxicillin 500 mg PO TID × 7 days. Local *E. coli* resistance: ciprofloxacin 250 mg PO BID × 3 days; levofloxacin 250 mg daily × 3 days; nitrofurantoin 100 mg PO BID × 7 days
- ▓ **Pyelonephritis:** oral or IV fluids, fever control, analgesic, antiemetic. UA/UCG pos cx. Outpt if stable, not toxic, and can keep down fluids; ceftriaxone 1 to 2 g IV followed by oral Abx. Ciprofloxacin 500 mg PO BID × 7 to 14 days; levofloxacin 750 mg PO daily × 5 days; amoxicillin 500 mg PO TID × 14 days; TMX/SMX (DS) 1 tab PO BID × 14 days; F/U 1 to 2 days. Admit for IV Abx if toxic, vomiting, refractory pain, comorbidities
  - ▓ Ciprofloxacin 400 mg IV BID; levofloxacin 750 mg IV QD; ceftriaxone 1 g IV QD
- ▓ **Balanitis/balanoposthitis:** FSBS, possible culture of discharge, retract foreskin and gentle cleansing, sitz baths, screen for STI, confirm ability to void. Clotrimazole 1% BID; miconazole 2% BID; nystatin cream BID; fluconazole 150 PO mg × 1; possible betamethasone 0.05% cream BID to decrease inflammation
  - ▓ Phimosis: topical steroids; urology referral
- ▓ **Paraphimosis:** analgesia, topical lubricant anesthetic, gentle continuous manual reduction; urology referral
- ▓ **Penile trauma:** analgesia, ice, elevate, UA, local wound care
- ▓ **Prostatitis:** UA and culture. Cipro 500 mg BID × 14 days or TMP/SMX (DS) 1 BID × 28 days
  High risk if urinary catheter or recent invasive procedure. Requires longer term Abx
  - ▓ **Suspect STI:** doxycycline 100 mg PO BID × 14 days plus ceftriaxone 250 mg IM; ciprofloxacin 500 mg PO BID × 14 days
  - ▓ **STI not suspected:** ciprofloxacin 500 mg PO BID × 2 to 3 weeks; levofloxacin 750 mg PO daily × 2 to 3 weeks; TMP/SMX (DS) 2 tabs PO BID × 28 days
  - ▓ If STIs are a concern, use Rocephin 250 mg IM × 1 *plus* doxycycline 100 mg BID × 14 days or Cipro 500 mg BID × 14 days
  - ▓ See www.cdc.gov/std/tg2015/default.htm
- ▓ **Torsion:** NSAIDs, opioids, antiemetic, elevate scrotum, maintain NPO. UA and culture. Confirm arterial blood flow by scrotal Doppler ultz. Emergent urology consult, manual detorsion, surgery
- ▓ **Epididymitis/Orchitis:** NSAIDs, analgesia, elevate scrotum, ice pack. UA (pyuria/bacteriuria), urine culture, urine GC/chlamydia, Gram stain if urethral discharge, possible CBC. Scrotal Doppler ultz to R/O torsion
  - ▓ **Suspect STI:** doxycycline 100 mg PO BID × 10 to 14 days plus ceftriaxone 250 mg IM; or if PCN allergic, azithromycin 2 g PO × 1
  - ▓ **STI not suspected:** ciprofloxacin 500 mg PO BID × 10 to 14 days or levofloxacin 750 PO daily × 10 to 14 days. Treat sexual partners

(cont.)

GENITOURINARY PROBLEMS (cont.)

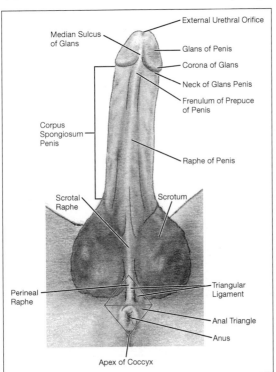

External Urethral Orifice

Median Sulcus of Glans

Glans of Penis

Corona of Glans

Neck of Glans Penis

Frenulum of Prepuce of Penis

Corpus Spongiosum Penis

Raphe of Penis

Scrotal Raphe

Scrotum

Perineal Raphe

Triangular Ligament

Anal Triangle

Anus

Apex of Coccyx

The external male genitalia

DICTATION/DOCUMENTATION

- **General:** alert, writhing, still, lethargic
- **VS and SaO$_2$:** fever, signs of shock
- **Skin:** PWD or pale, cool, moist; jaundice, dehydration
- **Abd:** flat, BSA, NT. No suprapubic tenderness or distension. No guarding or rebound
- **Back:** no CVAT to percussion
- **GU:**
  - **Male:** normal external genitalia circumcised/uncircumcised male; lesions or rash. Urinary meatus clear. Foreskin retracts easily. No scrotal erythema, warmth, tenderness, or skin breakdown. Testes normal in size and position. No fullness or tenderness over epididymis. No perineal tenderness or swelling
  - **Female:** normal external female genitalia, no blood in vaginal vault; no CMT; no uterine mass or tenderness, no adnexal fullness or TTP

(cont.)

GENITOURINARY PROBLEMS (cont.)

▶ TIPS

- Always obtain urine culture in older adults with UTI; however, a positive culture does not always indicate treatment if the pt is asymptomatic. Be cautious with treatment to prevent antibiotic resistance
- Review previous cultures and check renal function before Abx selection
- Monitor INR closely if on warfarin
- UTI in older males is less common and warrants close follow-up. An inflamed appendix may cause mild pyuria, hematuria, or proteinuria
- Normal exam findings suggest referred pain
- Direct hernia: through abd wall
- Indirect hernia: through inguinal canal
- Reversible causes of incontinence: DIAP:
  - D: delirium, dementia, depression
  - I: infection
  - A: atrophic vaginitis/urethritis. For atrophic vaginitis consider use of topical estrogen for a limited period of time
  - P: pharmaceuticals

DON'T MISS!

- Nitrofurantoin can cause severe confusion and agitation in some pts. Prescribe with caution for STI in males/females

USE OF URINARY CATHETER

Urinary catheterization is a commonly used and misused procedure, especially in the older adult. Catheters are sometimes placed for staff or pt convenience or comfort. However, CAUTI or complications related to the use of a urinary catheter are significant and increase daily as the catheter is in place. The catheter may cause discomfort or confusion in the older adult and lead to lack of mobility; older adult women are at highest risk for infection and increased mortality. Risks can be minimized by the use of specific indications for insertion and consideration of alternatives.

INDICATIONS

- Emergent testing needed such as altered mental status or urgent urologic procedure
- Close monitoring of urine output and unable to use a urinal or bedpan
- Urinary obstruction or retention
- Perineal or sacral open wound at risk for infection
- Too ill, fatigued, or incapacitated to use a bedpan or urinal; status after recent surgery
- Neurogenic bladder
- Hip or pelvic fracture
- Palliative or hospice care; management of incontinence requested by the pt or family

MANAGEMENT

- Must be inserted only by appropriately educated staff using strict aseptic technique
- Ensure that there is unobstructed urinary flow and catheter is anchored to minimize urethral irritation
- Remove the catheter as soon as possible

DICTATION/DOCUMENTATION

- The MDM should address the medical necessity for urinary catheter placement, clear indications for insertion, length of time, and when it will be removed

⊙ TIPS

- Consider alternative methods for urine collection such as an external catheter
- Incorporate surveillance program to monitor CAUTI

Sources: Adapted from Gould, C. (2017). *Catheter-associated urinary tract infection (CAUTI) toolkit.* Retrieved from https://www.cdc.gov/HAI/pdfs/toolkits/CAUTItoolkit_3_10.pdf; American College of Emergency Physicians, The American Geriatrics Society, Emergency Nurses Association, and the Society for Academic Emergency Medicine. (2013). *Geriatric emergency department guidelines.* Dallas, TX: American College of Emergency Physicians.

INCONTINENCE: BOWEL OR BLADDER

Fecal incontinence involves uncontrolled loss of the bowel for at least 1 month, which interferes with the pt's quality of life and requires some device to prevent soilage of clothing such as an adult diaper. It may cause social isolation.

FI can be caused by decreased sphincter tone, vaginal births that caused sphincter tears, damage from radiation treatment, fecal impaction, and idiopathic fecal incontinence.

Chronic diarrhea is diagnosed based on decrease in fecal consistency lasting more than 4 weeks.

Urinary incontinence involves the involuntary leakage of any amount of urine:
- Urge: uninhibited bladder contraction
- Stress: impaired urethral sphincter supports such as pelvic floor damage or failure of the sphincter caused by surgical damage. Mixed urge and stress
- Impaired bladder emptying caused by bladder obstruction (BPH) or detrusor underactivity from smooth muscle damage or diseases, such as diabetes mellitus, or neurologic damage, such as a spinal cord or disc herniation

HX
- Sudden or gradual onset
- Time: when does it occur? Before or after eating and/or drinking?
- GI: N/V, emesis: bloody, undigested food, bilious, projectile vomiting
- Constipation/diarrhea, bloody diarrhea, bowel changes, bloating, passing gas
- Flank pain, urinary urgency, frequency, burning pain, hematuria. Refusing or decreasing food or fluids
- Removing food from the mouth
- Diabetes
- Diverticular disease
- IBS
- *Clostridium difficile*
- Bladder prolapse
- Rectal prolapse
- Decreased sphincter tone from anal surgery, vaginal delivery, radiation proctitis
- Multiple UTI
- Previous urine cultures and treatment
- Medications (metformin, antibiotics)
- Laxative use

INCONTINENCE: BOWEL OR BLADDER (cont.)

PE

- **General:** alert and oriented, anxious, nervous, hyperactive
- **VS:** note vital signs and interpret as normal or abnormal, pulse ox interpretation, weight in kg (weight loss). Tachycardia or atrial arrhythmia. Systolic hypertension
- **Skin/Hair:** warm, dry, pink without rash. Good texture and turgor or smooth skin, inc perspiration, heat intolerance
- **HEENT:**
  - **Head:** normocephalic
  - **Eyes:** sclera and conjunctivae clear, PERRLA, EOMI, diplopia, proptosis, lid lag, stare
  - **Ears:** patent canals. Tympanic membranes clear. Dec hearing
  - **Nose/Face:** without rhinorrhea
  - **Mouth/Throat/Tongue:** mucous membranes are moist. Tongue symmetrical. Teeth present or absent. Posterior pharynx clear without erythema, lesions or exudate
- **Neck:** supple without meningismus or adenopathy, trachea midline. Carotids are equal. No bruits or jugular vein distention. No noted dysphagia or drooling
- **Chest:** normal AP diameter and no accessory muscle use noted. Good expansion without retractions. No tenderness. CTA, bilaterally with good tidal volume
- **Heart:** regular rate and rhythm (or tachycardia/AFib), no murmurs, rubs, or gallops; peripheral pulses present and equal. An S4 may be heard in healthy older people, which is suggestive of decreased ventricular compliance and impaired ventricular filling
- **Abd:** flat, soft, NT or protruding without masses, guarding, and rebound tenderness. BSA or hypoactive in all four quadrants. No hepatosplenomegaly
- **Back:** without spinal or CVA tenderness
- **Musculoskeletal:** limbs look longer in proportion to the trunk. Decreased tensile strength may be noted, caused by age or chronic disease such as osteoarthritis
- **GU:** normal external genitalia without lesions or masses. No hernia noted. Urinary continence or incontinence noted. **Female exam:** normal female genitalia, atrophic vaginal wall, presence or absence of a cystocele or rectocele. **Male external genitalia:** normal male genitalia, circumcised, uncircumcised, discharge
- **Pelvis/Hip:** nontender to palpation and stable to compression
- **Rectal:** normal tone or incontinent of stool. No rectal wall tenderness. Stool is brown and heme negative
- **Extremities:** FROM. Good to decreased strength bilaterally. Evidence of upper and lower extremity rigidity. No clubbing, cyanosis, or edema. Peripheral pulses intact, dorsalis pedal pulse may not be palpated, posterior tibial pulse present. Presence of vascular changes, varicose veins, vascular ulcers, pigmented skin, hair loss. Sensation intact or decreased. Hand tremor. Muscle weakness
- **Neuro:** alert, oriented or disoriented, dressed appropriately or signs of poor hygiene, such as lack of bathing, dirty hair and nails, clothes not clean, engaging, in no acute distress. Speech clear. Brief MME if indicated, that is, "What is the year, date, or month? Where are you—hospital or department?" Three-word recall. Cranial nerve II–XII intact. Motor sensory exam nonfocal. Moves all extremities. Gait: steady, unsteady. Romberg balance: normal or abnormal

(cont.)

INCONTINENCE: BOWEL OR BLADDER (cont.)

MDM/DDx

In spite of many specific etiologies for UI and FI, most pts are discharged home with a **nonspecific diagnosis.** Priority is on the early identification of pts with potentially life-threatening causes of UI and FI that can lead to sepsis or electrolyte abnormalities. Normal temperature, hemodynamic stability, and lack of serious comorbidities are reassuring findings. Consideration of extra-abd and bladder etiologies is important, including medications, **for example, metformin,** laxative use, and metabolic problems like **diabetes.** Diagnosis of **serious surgical problems, such as obstruction, intussusception, volvulus, strangulated hernia,** or **testicular torsion,** is vital. **Intractable pain, uncontrolled vomiting, unstable vital signs, or altered mental status, as well as altered electrolytes, such as hyponatremia,** in any pt are indications for hospital admission

MANAGEMENT

- Consider age, pain severity, hemodynamic stability, risk for serious etiology
- **High risk:** NPO, IV NS, analgesia, antiemetic
- **Labs:** CBC, elec, and creatinine, lactate level, lipase, UA Dip UA/UCG, FSBS. Recheck any pain, fluid tolerance, possible GC/chlamydia (**older adults are at great risk for STIs because they are not concerned about contraception**)
- **Imaging:** CXR: infiltrate, free air, KUB/abd, EKG, RUQ ultz; CT abd/pelvis
- Chronic UI and FI may require a referral to a specialist

DICTATION/DOCUMENTATION

- **General:** awake and alert, level of distress, anxiety, and in no acute distress
- **VS and SaO$_2$:** elevated temp, tachypnea, tachycardia
- **Skin:** PWD. No diaphoresis, cyanosis, or pallor
- **Abd:** flat without distension. No surface trauma, scars, incisions. BSA in all four quadrants. NT, guarding, rigidity to palpation. No tenderness, mass, pulsation in epigastric area. No organomegaly. Negative Murphy's sign. No periumbilical tenderness. No rebound in the lower quadrants. No tenderness over McBurney's point. Positive Murphy's sign. No suprapubic tenderness or distension. Good femoral pulses bilaterally. No hernia noted. No CVAT (include chest, GU, vaginal, rectal exam as indicated)
- **Rectal exam:** no fecal impaction noted
- **Vaginal exam:** vaginal atrophy, excoriation, discharge

ABDOMINAL X-RAY INTERPRETATION NOTE

If abd plain film ordered—document condition of aorta (e.g., calcification)

(cont.)

INCONTINENCE: BOWEL OR BLADDER (cont.)

⊙ TIPS

- Any leakage of stool or urine should be evaluated for the possibility of bowel or bladder infection
- Consider that changes in vaginal tissue may contribute to urinary problems
- Perform a pelvic exam on female pts with UI and/or FI to evaluate for bladder or rectal prolapse

DON'T MISS!

- Fecal incontinence at night
- Diarrhea that wakes the pt up at night

- Amount of urine in adult diapers and how often they are changed
- Fecal impaction when pt presents with chronic diarrhea and FI

LOW BACK PAIN

HX

- Onset, duration, intensity of pain; exact mechanism, such as fall, especially with axial load, prolonged sitting/standing, lifting, work related, stiffness in the morning
- Provoking, alleviating factors, such as pain increased with ambulation or improved by sitting or leaning forward. Prior back problems, workup, limitations, disability, pain management. Limitation in ROM/ambulation
- Quality and radiation of pain
- Motor or sensory changes, chronic or acute
- Pain begins abruptly then resolves or migrates to abd/back = TAD. Bowel or bladder retention or overflow incontinence
- Metastatic disease, weight loss, cough, pain worse at night F/C, N/V. Abd pain
- Urgency, frequency, dysuria, hematuria, HX of renal calculi. Pending litigation or sent by attorney
- HX: AAA/TAD, HTN, connective tissue disease (e.g., Marfan's syndrome), MI/ACS, CAD, hyperlipidemia, obesity, DM
- SH: smoker, ETOH, IVDA or illicit drug use

PE

- **General:** level of distress, appearance, nontoxic appearing
- **VS and SaO$_2$** (if indicated)
- **Skin:** PWD
- **Chest:** CTA bilaterally, no rales, rhonchi, or wheezing
- **Heart:** RRR, no murmurs, rubs, or gallops
- **Abd:** soft and NT without masses, guarding, or rebound. No epigastric tenderness or pulsatile mass. BSA. No HSM.
- **Back:** note gait to treatment area, symmetric, limp, antalgic, unable to bear weight, surface trauma, soft tissue or muscle tenderness, spasm, mass
    - PT tenderness, step-off, or deformity to palpation at midline CVAT/flank ecchymosis. SI notch tenderness, saddle anesthesia, anal wink, rectal tone
    - ROM—flexion/extension/lateral bending and rotation, note if limited or causes pain SLR—check for radiculopathy, sign if radiates below knee
    - Patellar reflexes: brisk, symmetric, muscle strength, lower extremities. Dorsiflexion/plantar flexion of ankles, heel/toe walk
    - Assess femoral pulses, possible rectal exam
- **Rectal:** tone, occult blood, melena
- **Extremities:** status of upper extremity circulation, femoral pulses, FROM, strength and sensation, weakness
- **Neuro:** A&O ×4, GCS, CN II–XII, no focal neuro deficit, DTRs, no pathological reflexes, gait steady, spontaneous or uncontrolled movements. Gait: Pt is or is not able to get up from a sitting position with or without assistance. Balance: steady, unsteady, use of an assistance device to ambulate. Romberg (check for pronator drift)

Nonorganic Etiology

- Pain with axial load on skull while standing
- Pain or sensory changes in nonanatomic distribution
- Flip test: Pt seated with legs dangling, told to steady self by holding edge of bed. Quickly flip up affected leg and pt will let go and fall back. Hold pt's wrists next to hips and turn body side to side to act like testing spinal rotation. No real stress on muscles or ligaments but pt complains of pain.

(cont.)

LOW BACK PAIN (cont.)

MDM/DDx

Serious causes more specific to the older adult include lumbar spinal stenosis, LS vertebral compression fractures, and issues related to bladder distention because of urinary retention. The majority of LBP caused by **an acute musculoskeletal injury or exacerbation** of a preexisting back/hip problem (**lumbar spondylolysis/spondylolisthesis, psoriatic arthritis, DDD, DJD, OA**). HX **osteoporosis,** >50 years, prolonged steroid use. Main focus is on potential **neurologic emergencies** or other than orthopedic etiology or complaints of pain such as **ACS or renal calculi.** Careful consideration of LBP "red flags" is an essential component of the examination. **Malignancy:** HX of tumor. **CA,** recent weight loss, pain >4 to 6 weeks, pain at night or at rest, ages >50 or <16 years. **Infection (discitis, transverse myelitis, epidural abscess** or **hematoma**): persistent fevers, IVDA, recent bacterial infections such as UTI or pyelonephritis, cellulitis, pneumonia. Immunosuppression from steroids, transplant, DM, HIV. Narrowing of the spinal canal is often worse in older adults and **spinal stenosis** can result in pain and neurological deficits. Pts often experience increased pain with standing associated with numbness and weakness often in both legs. **Cauda equina syndrome:** bilateral lower extremity pain, weakness, numbness; urinary retention followed by overflow; perineal or perianal anesthesia or poor rectal tone, progressive neurological deficits. **Herniation:** major muscle weakness (strength 3/5 or less), foot drop. **Trauma:** ejected from vehicle, fall from substantial height (e.g., **compression FXs**). **AAA/TAD:** atherosclerotic vascular disease, pain at night or rest, >60 years. Sudden, severe chest/abd pain radiating to the back/flank may indicate AAA/TAD. **Perforated viscus** may also cause acute LBP.

MANAGEMENT

- Thorough HX and PE to identify poss infectious or malignant etiology or suspected systemic disease
- Pain control: acetaminophen, NSAIDs, x-ray if MSK etiology
- TENS, opioids, alternate ice/heat for comfort. Encourage early mobility
- STAT EKG if suspect ACS
- Ultz for AAA/TAD
- Consider CBC, ESR, UA
- Imaging: plain LSpine x-rays are helpful in the older pt to look for DDD/DJD, vertebral compression FXs, spondylolisthesis, scoliosis, CA, and systemic diseases, such as osteoporosis and Paget disease; CT scan if bony pathology suspected
- MRI of spinal cord, disc herniation, or soft tissue etiology suspected
- Ortho/neuro referral for pain management, physical therapy, work tolerance evaluation, possible surg intervention

(cont.)

LOW BACK PAIN (cont.)

DICTATION/DOCUMENTATION

- **General:** level of distress
- **VS and SaO$_2$**
- **Skin:** PWD
- **Abd:** flat, BSA, NT to palp, no pulsatile masses, good femoral pulses
- **Back:** able to ambulate to treatment area with/without assistance, or arrived by wheelchair, stretcher, or ambulance. Seated/lying on the stretcher in no obvious/mild/moderate/severe distress. There is no surface trauma. Note abrasions, scars, ecchymosis, or lacerations if recent trauma. No STS or muscle, no spasm or mass, no point tenderness, step-off, or deformity of the bony cervical, thoracic, or LS spine to firm palpation at the midline. No CVA tenderness to percussion, no SI notch tenderness, no saddle anesthesia. ROM—able to stand erect. Normal flexion, extension, lateral bending, and rotation without limitation or complaint of pain (note degree of ROM). Heel and toe walk with good strength. Dorsi/plantar flexion with adequate/diminished strength. Straight leg raises are negative for radiculopathy. Note whether pain is increased in back, buttock, or radiation to what level of leg. Patellar reflexes equal and brisk bilaterally. Good dorsalis pedal pulses and posterior tibial pulse. Sensation to light touch is intact at the great toe web space. Normal anal wink or rectal tone

LUMBAR SPINE X-RAY INTERPRETATION NOTE

Lumbar spine x-ray interpretation: normal vertebral body and disc spaces. Normal spinal alignment, no evidence of spondylolisthesis. No obvious fracture or dislocation. No lytic lesions noted. SI joints appear normal

❍ TIPS

- *Neuro Status*
    - L3 = extend quad or do deep knee bend/sensation lateral thigh
    - L4 = dorsiflexion ankle or heel walk/sensation medial thigh and ankle
    - L5 = dorsiflexion great toe or toe walk/sensation lateral leg and dorsum foot
    - S1 = stand on toes/sensation lateral ankle and sole of foot, ankle jerk reflex
- *Reflexes*
    - 0 = no reflex
    - 1 = hyporeflexia
    - 2 = normal
    - 3 = hyperreflexia
    - 4 = clonus

(cont.)

LOW BACK PAIN (cont.)

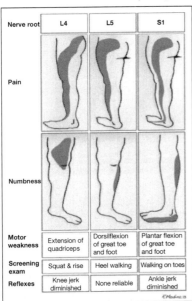

Nerve root	L4	L5	S1
Pain			
Numbness			
Motor weakness	Extension of quadriceps	Dorsiflexion of great toe and foot	Plantar flexion of great toe and foot
Screening exam	Squat & rise	Heel walking	Walking on toes
Reflexes	Knee jerk diminished	None reliable	Ankle jerk diminished

Testing for lumbar nerve root compromise

TIPS FOR EXAMINING THE OLDER ADULT

Physical Exam Findings	Etiology
Asymmetric range of motion of the LS spine	Mechanical disc disease
Spinal tenderness	Compression Fracture Infection
Weakness of L4–L5 and L5–S1 muscles	Mechanical disc disease, lumbar spinal stenosis
Normal spinal exam	Osteoporotic sacral fracture, hip disease, tumor Referred visceral pain

Source: Adapted from Flaherty, E., & Resnick, B. (Eds.). (2014). *Geriatric nursing review syllabus: A core curriculum in advanced practice geriatric nursing* (4th ed.). New York, NY: American Geriatrics Society.

(cont.)

LOW BACK PAIN (cont.)

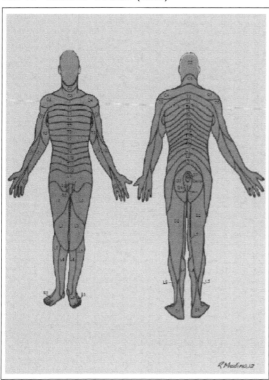

Dermatomes diagram

UPPER EXTREMITY (SHOULDER, ELBOW, WRIST PAIN/INJURY)

HX

- Onset, location, and degree of pain
- MOI: FOOSH, fall directly on elbow or shoulder, assault, MVC; consider syncope.
- Duration/type of pain—sharp, throbbing, constant, intermittent. Characteristics— (e.g., hand: "fullness," throbbing pain, swelling of fingertips)
- Aggravating factors/relieving factors/treatments—OTC meds, immobilization
- Recent illness/infection
- F/C, redness, warmth, STS, streaking
- ROM limitations, exacerbation/radiation of pain; numbness or tingling, weak grip
- Other joint involvement
- Occupation/work injury
- Hand dominance
- Previous illness or injury or surgical intervention to upper extremity
- OA/RA; gout/pseudogout
- Calcium pyrophosphate dihydrate deposition disease (CPPD)
- Animal or human bite/high pressure puncture injury (see "Wounds/Lacerations")

PE

- **General**: level of distress
- **VS and SaO$_2$** (if indicated) compare entire upper extremity with unaffected side
- **Pain** level (e.g., out of proportion to injury, consider compartment syndrome)
- **Pallor** (skin color)
- **Pulses** (distal pulses/cap refill)
- **Poikilothermic** (compare with surrounding temp)
- **Paralysis** (ROM)/strength/grip, paresthesias (sensation)
- **Puffiness** (swelling)
- **Pressure** (tenseness—smoothness of skin), compartment syndrome
- **Position** of limb (e.g., angulated)
- **Nerves: ulnar nerve**: abduct fingers against resistance, sensation on ulnar surface little finger
- **Median nerve**: oppose thumb and little finger, enervates palmar surface of thumb, index, middle, and half of the ring finger and thenar eminence
- **Radial nerve**: extend wrist and fingers against resistance, sensation on dorsal web space between thumb and index finger
- **Include HEENT, neck, chest wall, lungs, and spine as indicated: high index of suspicion for associated injury in older adults**

PROXIMAL HUMERUS

- STS, surface trauma, ecchymosis (may be extensive and involve chest wall or back), hematoma, open wound, obvious wound, deformity, position, prominent humeral head. Bony step-off or crepitus or muscle weakness. Assess sensation over lateral deltoid; ROM of shoulder, elbow, wrist; intact radial and ulnar pulses and cap refill. Reassess for increasing swelling or pulsatile hematoma caused by vascular injury
- Assess elbow, wrist, hand

(cont.)

UPPER EXTREMITY (SHOULDER, ELBOW, WRIST PAIN/INJURY) (cont.)

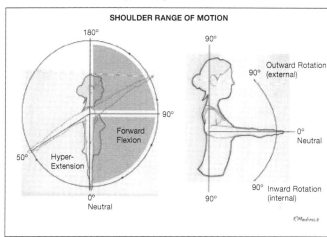

SHOULDER RANGE OF MOTION

The shoulder range of motion

DISTAL HUMERUS/ELBOW
- STS, surface trauma, ecchymosis, open wounds, obvious deformity (may be very unstable), position. Local TTP over medial or lateral epicondyle, olecranon, radial head, or distal bicep
- Assess motor/sensory function of radial, median, ulnar nerves. Intact brachial, radial, ulnar pulses, and cap refill. Avoid ROM to avoid neurovascular damage. Focal STS, TTP, erythema, bogginess over olecranon. Assess shoulder, wrist, hand

WRIST
- STS, surface trauma, open wounds. TTP over distal radius, distal ulna, scaphoid, ulnar styloid (to compression or axial load). Feeling of fullness or obvious deformity
- Motor/sensory function of ulnar, median, radial nerves. Distal motor/neurovascular status. Intact radial and ulnar pulses and cap refill. ROM: flex/ext, ulnar/radial deviation. Phalen's or Tinel's sign (carpal tunnel syndrome), Finkelstein test (De Quervain's tenosynovitis)
- Assess shoulder, elbow

(cont.)

UPPER EXTREMITY (SHOULDER, ELBOW, WRIST PAIN/INJURY) (cont.)

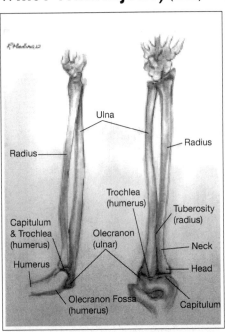

Anatomy of the elbow

(cont.)

UPPER EXTREMITY (SHOULDER, ELBOW, WRIST PAIN/INJURY) (cont.)

MDM/DDx

Upper extremity injuries in the older adult population are common and can be associated with significant morbidity and functional impairment. Loss of independence and ability to care for self are frequent sequelae. Even low-impact falls can cause serious injury especially in osteoporotic older women. **Proximal humerus FXs** are often associated with **axillary nerve damage, brachial plexus nerve palsy** or **axillary arterial injuries** are much less common. **Rotator cuff injury** must be considered in all proximal humerus FXs. An elevated anterior fat pad or any visible posterior fat pad indicates the presence of an **elbow FX** even if not clear on x-ray. FXs involving the **distal humerus FXs** are less common but can have significant swelling; damage to the brachial artery can lead to vascular compromise; **compartment syndrome** is a serious complication. Clinical suspicion of FX based on examination should require conservative management with splint and reevaluation. Older adults may have elbow pain from **olecranon bursitis** associated with gout and RA. **Wrist FX** is very common in older adults and is often intra-articular; severity is also based on degree of angulation or displacement. Hyperextension mechanism should prompt evaluation of **scaphoid fracture**, a common and easily missed carpal fracture. Most scaphoid fractures involve the narrow waist of the bone; compromised blood flow to the proximal portion of the bone can lead to **avascular necrosis**. Assessment of the alignment and **lunate–capitate** relationship is vital in the consideration of rare but serious **lunate** or **perilunate dislocations.** These injuries are most often associated with a history of extreme flexion or extension of the wrist. **Soft tissue injuries**, such as **sprains or tendonitis**, can also cause prolonged pain or instability. **Carpal tunnel syndrome** results in compressive neuropathy of the median nerve and presents with burning and numbness of the volar surface of the first three digits. Repetitive lifting can lead to **De Quervain's tenosynovitis**, entrapment of the tendons of the wrist causing pain during thumb flexion. Other causes of falls in older adults include **ACS** or **dysrhythmias, CVA, and intracranial etiology**

MANAGEMENT

- General: immobilize in a sling or splint, rest, ice, elevation, analgesia-NSAIDs; Abx for open FXs
- Consider: FSBS, baseline labs EKG, noncontrast head CT if possible syncope
- Immediate consult for neurovascular injuries, compartment syndrome amputations; severe FXs/dislocation, consult

PROXIMAL HUMERUS

- X-ray: AP and lateral in axial or Y view. FXs of humeral neck and greater tuberosity are common. Suspect shoulder dislocation if glenohumeral joint not clearly visible. Axial view is helpful to identify fragments. CT helpful in evaluation of articular involvement
- Urgent reduction of shoulder dislocations
- Vascular surgical consultation if concern for limb ischemia
- Most are minimally displaced; initial management of stable FXs is immobilization with a sling or sling and swath

(cont.)

UPPER EXTREMITY (SHOULDER, ELBOW, WRIST PAIN/INJURY) (cont.)

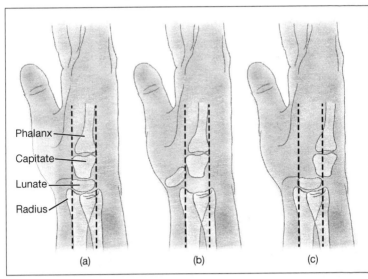

(a) Normal wrist, (b) lunate, and (c) perilunate dislocations

DISTAL HUMERUS/ELBOW

- X-ray: AP and lateral, may include forearm. Look for elevated fat pads caused by joint effusion; visible anterior fat pad may be normal but visible posterior fat pad always indicates fracture. Assess anterior humeral and radiocapitellar lines. CT/MRI usually not indicated acutely
- Doppler or angiography is concern for vascular integrity; vascular surgical consultation
- Long arm or coaptation (double sugar tong) posterior splint; elbow 90 and forearm neutral
- Nonoperative conservative management with sling and/or cast is appropriate for many older adults especially with comorbidities, dementia, or those who are not surgical candidates
- Olecranon bursitis: compression, avoid local pressure or trauma, possible aspiration but risk of reaccumulation

WRIST

- X-ray: lateral view most helpful, also obtain AP and oblique views. Carpal bones are in two rows; joint spaces are all 1 to 2 mm wide (if wider, suspect ligamentous injury). Nondisplaced impacted FX may only show as a slight whitish line because of overlapping bone density. Scaphoid FX may be subtle and missed or not visualized on x-ray; obtain navicular view if suspicion high for FX. Capitate, lunate, and radius articulate in a straight line; look for lunate or perilunate dislocation. Look for associated ulnar styloid FX. Distal fragment displacement: posterior = Colles' FX; anterior = Smith's FX. CT may be indicated for scaphoid, lunate, or capitate FXs
- Closed reduction and immobilization of stable FXs. Thumb spica splint and close follow-up for suspected scaphoid FX

(cont.)

UPPER EXTREMITY (SHOULDER, ELBOW, WRIST PAIN/INJURY) (cont.)

DICTATION/DOCUMENTATION

- ▓ **General:** level of distress
- ▓ **VS and SaO$_2$** (if indicated)
- ▓ **Skin:** PWD, normal texture and turgor
- ▓ **HEENT:** (as indicated)
- ▓ **Neck:** no point tenderness, step-off, or deformity to firm palpation of the midline posterior cervical spine. Full flexion, extension, lateral bending, and rotation without limitation or complaint of pain. No soft tissue swelling, spasm, or TTP
- ▓ **Extremities:** the R/L shoulder/elbow/wrist/hand is with/without obvious asymmetry or deformity when compared to the R/L. No surface trauma or open wounds, STS, ecchymosis, or open, obvious deformity. No bony deformity, crepitus, or focal area of TTP. Distal motor and neurovascular status are intact. No overlying erythema or warmth (nontrauma)
- ▓ **Include specific areas as indicated (following)**
  - ▓ **Proximal humerus:** no prominence or TTP of the humeral head, no TTP over the clavicle, A–C joint, acromion, or scapula. No tenderness to palpation of the bicipital groove or soft tissues. No pain or limitation with active or passive abduction/adduction, internal/external rotation, flexion/extension. Normal sensation over the deltoid and ability to flex arm at elbow indicates intact axillary nerve function
  - ▓ **Elbow:** no bony tenderness to palpation of the lateral or medial epicondyle, olecranon, or radial head. Normal flexion, extension, supination, and pronation. Normal muscle strength. Intact motor and sensation of ulnar, median, and radial nerves.
  - ▓ No epicondylar or axillary lymphadenopathy. No focal STS, erythema, warmth, or fluctuance over olecranon. No joint irritability
  - ▓ **Wrist:** no scaphoid fullness or TTP to direct palpation or axial load. Normal flex/ext, ulnar/radial deviation. Motor/sensory function of ulnar, radial, and median nerves intact. Ulnar and radial pulses intact. Negative Phalen's/Tinel's sign (carpal tunnel syndrome). Negative Finkelstein test (De Quervain's tenosynovitis)

X-RAY NOTE

For example, a _____ x-ray series was performed. There was no fracture, dislocation, soft tissue swelling, or foreign body noted (For the wrist, dictate that normal joint spaces were seen.)

SPLINT NOTE

There was no neurovascular compromise after splint/sling application; the splint was in good alignment and the pt had good sensation and capillary refill at the time of discharge

SHOULDER REDUCTION PROCEDURE NOTE

Procedure explained and consent obtained. Procedural sedation protocol was followed per institutional protocol and the L/R shoulder was successfully reduced by performing external rotation, Stimson, scapular manipulation, or traction/counter traction. Neurovascularly intact following procedure; sling and swathe applied after postreduction x-ray demonstrates complete reduction. Tolerated procedure well with no complications

(cont.)

UPPER EXTREMITY (SHOULDER, ELBOW, WRIST PAIN/INJURY) (cont.)

DISTAL HUMERUS

- Elevated anterior fat pad ("sail sign") or any visible posterior fat pad
- Badly displaced, or intra-articular FX
- Peripheral nerve injury (median nerve) with supracondylar FX
- Neurovascular impairment (brachial nerve with humeral FX; ulnar nerve with olecranon FX)
- Significant STS or risk for compartment syndrome

WRIST

- Nondisplaced impacted distal radius FX
- Navicular/scaphoid FX—most commonly injured carpal bone, easily missed, can lead to avascular necrosis
- Lunate or perilunate dislocations

❯ SHOULDER TIPS

- **AC separation:** pain over joint, possible high-riding bony deformity palpable or visible on x-ray
- **Rotator cuff tear:** anterolateral pain referred to deltoid, limited abduction, and internal rotation; drop arm test; empty can test
- **Bicipital tendonitis:** pain over bicipital groove, by shoulder flexion, forearm supination, and/or elbow flexion
- Local steroid injection for pain management for shoulder pain in the older adult when it is not an acute injury

❯ ELBOW TIPS

- **X-ray:** good lateral film is essential; "figure 8" or hourglass sign at distal humerus. Fat pad elevation: anterior "sail sign" or any visible posterior fat pad is abnormal even if no fracture seen
- **Document suspected occult FX:** splint or sling for conservative management. Refer for repeat x-ray in 7 to 10 days
- **Ortho referral:** displaced, unstable, open, or intra-articular FXs; FX >30% radial head; FX >3 mm or 30° displaced

❯ WRIST TIP

- Thumb spica splint and close follow-up for suspected scaphoid FX to prevent AVN

DON'T MISS!

Proximal humerus

- C-spine injury
- Pneumothorax
- Peripheral nerve injury
- Vascular injury

HAND PAIN/INJURY

HX

- MOI: work or sports related, hyperextension/flexion, crush, forceful abduction of thumb
- Animal or human bite
- High-pressure puncture injury
- Movement limitations
- Feeling of fullness, throbbing pain, burning
- Swelling of fingertip, erythema, proximal lymphangitis
- Occupation, hand dominance
- Work-related injury
- Onset, duration, delayed
- Presentation pain, F/C
- OA/RA
- Calcium pyrophosphate
- Dihydrate deposition disease
- CPPD (pseudogout)

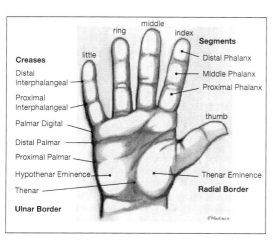

Palmar surface of the hand

(cont.)

HAND PAIN/INJURY (cont.)

PE
- **General**: level of distress
- **VS and SaO$_2$** (if indicated)
- **Upper extremity—hand/fingers**
- **Note**: compare with unaffected side; examine open wounds under good light with bloodless field; include range of motion and movement against resistance and repeat under anesthesia
- Color, temperature, ecchymosis, open wound, bleeding, erythema, warmth, exudate
- Note local or diffuse STS or fusiform swelling of digit, Heberden's (DIP joint) or Bouchard's (PIP joint) nodes, TTP, bony step-off, crepitus, or deformity, sensation to light touch. Pulses and capillary refill, distal neurovascular status FROM, including isolated FDS/FDP of each digit
- Normal cascade of fingers, no malrotation (all fingers point toward scaphoid)
- **Examine**: shoulder, elbow, hand/fingers

FLEXOR TENDONS
- FDS and FDP

EXTENSOR TENDONS
- **Abductor pollicis longus and extensor pollicis brevis:** abduct thumb from other fingers
- **Extensor carpi radialis longus and extensor carpi radialis brevis:** make fist and extend hand at wrist
- **Extensor pollicis longus:** with the palm down, patient should be able to raise the thumb
- **Extensor carpi ulnaris:** ulnar deviation, intact extension of digits against resistance
- **Ligaments:** ulnar collateral ligament of thumb has strong opposition

NERVES
- **Ulnar nerve:** abduct fingers against resistance, sensation on ulnar surface of little finger
- **Median nerve:** oppose thumb and little finger, enervates palmar surface of thumb, index, middle, and half of the ring finger
- **Radial nerve:** extend wrist and fingers against resistance, sensation on dorsal web space between thumb and index finger

NAILS
- Nail avulsion, tissue avulsion, partial/complete amputation, subungual hematoma

MD/DDx
Older adults may experience a burning sensation in the hands in spite of a normal exam and causes for **neuritis**, such as diabetes or alcohol or **vitamin B deficiency**, should be considered. Edema of the hands may be related to **hypoproteinuria** or **anasarca** caused by hepatic, renal, or cardiac disease. Infections of the fingers and hand include local **paronychia**, **felon**, **cellulitis**, and **flexor tenosynovitis**. Soft tissue injuries, such as minor sprains, are usually benign. More serious injuries involve the volar plate or lateral collateral ligament. Extensor tendon damage can result in permanent deformity such as a **mallet finger** or **Boutonniere deformity**. Strength and function of the FDS and FDP against resistance evaluates the **flexor tendons**. **Dislocated digits** should be reduced promptly and concurrent FX considered. Orthopedic consultation is needed if unable to reduce an FX, **unstable FXs** that involve >25% of the articular surface, **unstable ligamentous injury**, or potential serious **closed space infection** of a finger or hand. **Carpal tunnel syndrome** is suggested by progressive burning pain in the distribution of the median nerve

(cont.)

HAND PAIN/INJURY (cont.)

MANAGEMENT

- **Paronychia**: warm soaks, NSAIDs. Use #10 scalpel or blunt instrument to "sweep" and elevate nail fold to promote drainage. Keep open with wick of packing gauze. Hot soaks. No Abx. Consider felon, herpetic whitlow
- **Felon**: x-ray if concern for osteomyelitis or FB. Digital block and decompress with vertical incision over volar distal phalanx, which is least likely to cause damage. Pack loosely, splint. Abx as for cellulitis or antiviral if herpes suspected (do not I&D)
- **Flexor tenosynovitis**: culture discharge, including fungal, possible CBC, ESR, x-ray. Analgesia, splint in POF. ABX cefazolin 1 to 2 g IV QID; clindamycin 600 to 900 mg IV TID. Ampicillin/sulbactam 1.5 to 3 g IV QID if immunosuppressed or bite wound
- **Mallet finger**: analgesia, x-ray, splint DIP joint in full extension for 6 weeks
- **Boutonniere deformity**: analgesia, x-ray, splint PIP joint in full extension for 6 weeks. **Ulnar collateral ligament injury (gamekeeper's or skier's thumb)**: thumb spica splint
- **Tendon injuries**: lacerations over a tendon can sometimes be loosely approximated, the hand immobilized, prophylactic Abx given, and referred for surgical repair

DICTATION/DOCUMENTATION

- **General**: level of distress
- **VS and SaO$_2$** (if indicated)
- **Hand/Fingers**: the R/L hand is without obvious asymmetry or deformity compared to the R/L hand. No swelling, erythema, atrophy, or obvious deformity. No surface trauma, open wounds, nail avulsion, tissue avulsion, partial or complete amputation, subungual hematoma, or bony deformity. Normal cascade of fingers. Normal flexion and extension of the fingers. FDS and FDP intact against resistance. No focal fullness, throbbing pain, swelling of fingertip
- NT to palpation—describe exact joint, digit, or location. Pulses and cap refill

○ TIPS

Consider flexor tendon involvement in any trauma to forearm, palm, or digits
- **Neuro level**
- **C6** = palmar surface of thumb, index, 1/2 of the third finger
- **C7** = palmar surface third finger
- **C8** = palmar surface of fourth and fifth fingers

X-RAY NOTE

There was no fracture, dislocation, soft tissue swelling, or foreign body noted

SPLINT NOTE

There was no neurovascular compromise after splint application; the splint was in good alignment and the pt had good sensation and capillary refill at the time of discharge

DON'T MISS!

Flexor tendon injury	Compartment syndrome
Vascular injuries	High-pressure penetration

(cont.)

HAND PAIN/INJURY (cont.)

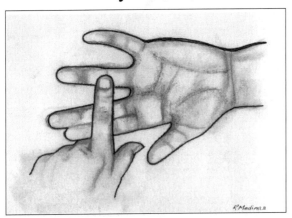

Assessment of flexor digitorum profundus (FDP)
Note: Hold middle phalanx in complete extension and evaluate the
strength of **flexion of the distal phalanx (DIP)**. Repeat for each digit.

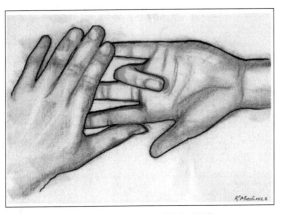

Assessment of flexor digitorum superficialis (FDS)
Note: Hold nonaffected digits in complete extension and evaluate
the strength of flexion of the PIP joint with the DIP joints in
extension. It is important to eliminate the use of intrinsic palmar
muscles in order to isolate the flexor tendon.

HIP/PELVIC INJURY

HX

- Onset, duration, MOI, LOC, neck, back pain
- Consider syncope, cardiac, neuro etiology for fall
- Able to get up and bear weight after injury; length of time on ground
- Urge but inability to void
- Hear or feel snap or pop, pain related to activities
- Other areas of pain: head, neck, back
- HX of OA/RA

PE

- **General**: level of distress
- **VS and SaO$_2$:** tachycardia, hypotension, signs of shock
- **Skin:** PWD, cool, pale, moist
- **Note:** complete head-to-toe exam for occult injuries (see "Trauma Template")
- **Pelvis:** surface trauma, TTP over symphysis pubis, pubic rami, ischial bone, iliac crest, barrel hoop sign compression. Abduct/adduction of hip
- **Hip:** compare with unaffected side, obvious asymmetry, deformity/crepitus. Int or ext rotation or shortening, STS, surface trauma, ecchymosis, open wounds deformity/crepitus, position, painful abduction
    - TTP over greater trochanter, SI notch, buttocks, quadriceps, femoral triangle, inguinal area
    - Femoral pulses, distal neurovascular status. Intertrochanteric FX: leg shortened and ext rotated
    - Greater trochanter FX: painful to palp, especially with abduction but may not have obvious deformity
    - Lesser trochanter FX: pain with flexion and internal rotation. Femoral neck FX; severe pain, slight shortening, abducted and ext rotated. Subtrochanteric FX: proximal femur flexed and ext rotation
- **GU:** blood at urinary meatus, gross hematuria, perineal ecchymosis, high-riding prostate distended bladder, inability to void (risk for concomitant bladder, urethral, or rectal injury)

MDM/DDx

Falls affect 2/3 of people over 65 years and are often associated with other serious injuries. Contributing factors are often decreased mobility and strength, dizziness, cognitive impairment, and poor vision. Older adults, especially osteoporotic females, are at risk for **pelvic FX** from even minor falls. In general, they have a poorer outcome than younger pts often related to hemorrhage, TBI, or subsequent multisystem organ failure. The incidence of **hip FX** also increases significantly as people age and is associated with substantial morbidity and mortality. MDM for hip/pelvic injuries includes a high index of suspicion and search for concomitant injuries. Intertrochanteric and subtrochanteric FXs are at higher risk for hemorrhage. All hip fractures must be evaluated based on the anatomic location, inherent risk factors, and need for operative intervention.

(cont.)

HIP/PELVIC INJURY (cont.)

MANAGEMENT

- ABCs
- Venous access and volume resuscitation as indicated, analgesia
- Avoid excessive movement of hip/pelvis; support with pillows; traction splint/pelvic binder
- Analgesia
- Maintain NPO for possible surgical repair
- **Labs:** CBC, serial H&H (monitor blood loss), chem panel, coags, type and cross if indicated, UA (hematuria)
- **Imaging:**
  - X-rays: AP pelvis x-ray will identify most pelvic FXs. Check film carefully for more than one FX of pelvic ring. Plain films may underestimate symphysis pubic deformity because of associated muscle spasm
  - AP and lateral hip x-rays also show most FXs but a complete pelvis should be included to rule out pubic rami FX and allow comparison of both hips. Preoperative pelvic angiograms are recommended for fractures involving the greater sciatic notch
  - Ultz: abd FAST scan if intraperitoneal bleeding is suspected
  - CT in major trauma pts; helpful to evaluate acetabular FXs with posterior hip dislocation, MRI is helpful in identifying FXs in pts with negative x-rays but index of suspicion is high. Retrograde urethrogram if urethral injury suspected

CONSULTATION AND ADMISSION

Urgent orthopedic consultation for surgical management of femoral neck FXs, intertrochanteric hip FXs that are common in older adult populations, and most tension femoral neck stress FXs require surgical intervention. Symphysis pubis disruptions are stabilized operatively with external fixation (6–12 weeks) and may require ORIF if unstable. Pubic ramus FXs must be evaluated for associated injury to urinary bladder, vagina, and perineum and may require surgery. Iliac wing FXs and posterior iliac fragment FXs often also require definitive surgical repair. Sacroiliac joint disruptions are usually managed nonoperatively with external fixators. Sacral FXs occur with pelvic ring injuries and are usually treated by indirect reduction techniques

DICTATION/DOCUMENTATION

- **General:** level of distress
- **VS and SaO$_2$** (see "Trauma Dictation")
- **Hip/Pelvis:** Pt is able to ambulate to treatment area with/without difficulty or assistance, pain, limp, or antalgic gait. No surface trauma or ecchymosis. No erythema or warmth. No deformity, crepitus, or obvious asymmetry of the affected leg compared to the other leg. No TTP over symphysis pubis, ischial bone, iliac crest, trochanter, SI notch, buttocks, quadriceps, femoral triangle, or inguinal ligament. No inguinal lymphadenopathy. ROM unlimited and without pain. Normal flexion to chest (135°), extension (30°), abduction (45°), adduction across midline, internal/external rotation (45°). Distal motor and neurovascular status are intact

(cont.)

HIP/PELVIC INJURY (cont.)

X-RAY NOTE

There was no fracture, dislocation, soft tissue swelling, or foreign body noted

SPLINT NOTE

There was no neurovascular compromise after splint application; the splint was in good alignment and the pt had good sensation and capillary refill at the time of discharge

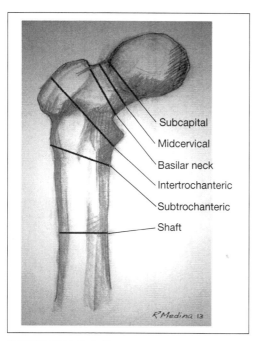

Common hip fracture sites

(cont.)

HIP/PELVIC INJURY (cont.)

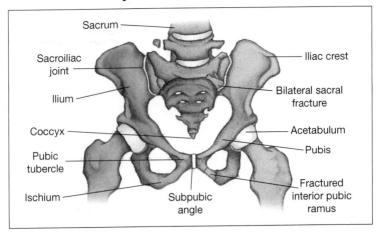

Sacrum

Sacroiliac joint

Ilium

Coccyx

Pubic tubercle

Ischium

Subpubic angle

Iliac crest

Bilateral sacral fracture

Acetabulum

Pubis

Fractured interior pubic ramus

The anatomy of the pelvis

⊙ TIPS

- Explore cause and consult with internal medicine for underlying issues and clearance for surgical intervention
- One pelvis FX often associated with another FX
- Most pelvis FXs are stable (single ischial ramus, unilateral FXs both rami, iliac wing)
- Unstable pelvic FXs involve both anterior and posterior arches (double break in pelvic ring) or widened symphysis pubis with SI joint disruption even if no FX seen
- **Impacted hip FX may only be seen as a subtle white line**
- If unable to bear weight, consider CT/MRI of hip for occult FX. If unable to bear weight—crutches, then recheck 1 to 2 days

DON'T MISS!

- Many older adults often have other comorbidities (vertigo/syncope, cardiac arrhythmias, dehydration, med issues)
- Intra-abd or pelvic etiology
- Syncope or underlying medical condition as reason for injury

KNEE PAIN

HX

- Onset, duration, redness, pain, F/C, STS immediate/gradual, ability to bear weight, MOI—direct trauma, foot planted/knee twisted; fall on flexed knee (tibial plateau FX)
- Locking—unable to move passively, 45° flexed (meniscus or cruciate injury); clicking, crepitus, or feeling of giving way (ACL injury)
- HX patellar or knee joint dislocation/reduction
- OA/RA, gout, pseudogout (calcium pyrophosphate disease)

PE

- **General**: level of distress
- **VS and SaO$_2$** (if indicated)
- **Lower extremity—knee**
- **Note**: compare with unaffected side, observe gait and ability to bear weight. Exam often difficult because of pain and swelling. Perform knee exam with pt supine; visualize both legs from the groin to toes and compare. Obvious asymmetry, deformity/crepitus, patella location, STS/effusion, surface trauma, ecchymosis, open wounds, position, erythema, warmth, joint irritability TTP over patella, lat/med joint line prox fibula, popliteal pulse/fullness. ROM: flex/ext, able to do deep knee bend with symmetry (130°), fully extend knee, internal and external rotation (10°)
- Laxity with valgus or varus stress. Distal motor/neurovascular status
- **Effusion**: <6 hours with cruciate lig, meniscus, FX. Slower onset and recurrent effusion more likely with meniscus injury. Patella ballottement.
- **Tibial sag**: flex 90° and see if tibia sags posteriorly
- **Lachman/Drawer maneuver**
- **McMurray/Apley compression test**
- **Examine:** back, hip, ankle, and foot

(cont.)

KNEE PAIN (cont.)

MDM/DDx

Most people experience knee pain at some point in life and the incidence increases with age. Focus is on differentiating between intra-articular and extra-articular causes of knee pain. Internal problems include **OA, RA,** or **inflammatory arthritis, gout, infection, tendonitis/ bursitis,** or **structural changes.** Knee pain can also be caused by pain referred from the **hip** or **low back**. **OA** is common as a result of degenerative changes as the knee ages. It is often seen in women and the obese, who complain of gradually worsening ache, stiffness, and swelling. **RA** is an uncommon chronic autoimmune condition that leads to damage of the synovial lining and joint inflammation. Pts complain of pain and morning stiffness with swelling and limited ROM; extra-articular findings may include rash and symmetrical joint involvement. **Gout** and **pseudogout** are crystal-induced arthropathies. Gout is caused by uric acid that accumulates and crystallizes in synovial joints causing sudden severe pain, swelling, and redness. Although gout usually affects the great toe or ankle, it can also affect the knee. It is more common in older men, often precipitated by alcohol, purine rich foods (seafood, poultry, meat), diuretics, or stress. Calcium pyrophosphate crystals cause pseudogout but presenting symptoms are similar in each disease. It is important to distinguish gout or pseudogout from an acute knee joint infection and requires joint aspiration. Acute gout may also present as cellulitis. **Septic joints** are usually associated with fever and malaise in addition to a red, warm, swollen knee. Consider prosthesis involvement and possibility of gonococcal organism, especially if more than one joint affected. Failure to diagnosis an infected joint can lead to significant morbidity and mortality. **Patellar** or **tibial plateau FXs** may require surgical intervention. Consider ruptured **Baker's cyst** or **DVT** in cases of posterior knee pain. Internal derangement injuries usually result in an effusion. **Meniscus tear** usually presents with JLT, pain with weight bearing, + McMurray test, locking, or giving way. ACL injury is associated with immediate severe pain, "popping" sensation, instability, +Lachman/drawer tests, unable to ambulate. **PCL tear** is an uncommon injury that results from a fall on a flexed knee or direct trauma to the front of the knee. Other causes of knee pain to consider include **prepatellar bursitis** (TTP over patella, swelling and redness over infrapatellar area, and inability to flex or put pressure on knee)

(cont.)

KNEE PAIN (cont.)

MANAGEMENT

- **OA**: rest, ice, careful short-term use of NSAIDs and analgesia. Encourage weight loss and exercise. Ortho referral for severe cases
- **RA/Inflammatory**: ice/heat therapy, supportive splints, analgesics, poss steroids and joint aspiration. Rheumatology referral for labs and initiation of disease-modifying antirheumatic drugs (DMARDs)
- **Gout**: consider septic joint. NSAIDs, including indomethacin, analgesia, steroids
- Avoid alcohol and high-purine foods. Colchicine 1.2 mg PO, followed by 0.6 mg in 1 hour (review renal/hepatic function and recent meds for contraindications)
- **Septic joint**: prompt identification of infection by joint aspiration and analysis. WBC >50,000 PMN but may be less. Parenteral Abx, analgesia, immobilization. Abx choice and duration are dictated based on specific organism involved. Vancomycin 15 to 20 mg/kg BID plus ceftriaxone 2 g QD or ciprofloxacin 400 mg TID. Infected prosthetic joint—rifampin 600 mg QD after consultation
- **Tendonitis/bursitis**: NSAIDs, analgesia, ice, immobilize
- **Trauma:**
  - **Patellar dislocation**: manual reduction for simple horizontal dislocation (lateral most common). Place pt supine, extend knee with gentle, anteromedial pressure over lateral patella to lift patella over femoral condyle. Use knee immobilizer, crutches
  - **Knee dislocation**: assess for vascular injury and immediate reduction, emergent ortho and/or vascular consult
  - **Tibial plateau FX**: NSAIDs, analgesia, ice, immobilize, x-ray. Knee immobilizer, crutches with nonweight bearing if FX is nondisplaced or only minimally (4–10 mm) displaced. Surgery needed if open, significantly displaced, or depressed. Consider compartment syndrome

DICTATION/DOCUMENTATION

- **General**: level of distress
- **VS and SaO$_2$**
- **Knee**: pt is able to bear weight and ambulate without pain. No surface trauma, STS, or obvious effusion. No overlying erythema or warmth (medical complaints). There is no obvious asymmetry or deformity when the R/L knee is compared with R/L knee. Pt is able to perform deep knee bend with symmetry (130°), fully extend knee, and perform internal and external rotation (10°). No tenderness to palpation of the patella, no effusion or ballottement. No tenderness over the infrapatellar tendon or bursa. No tenderness over the medial or lateral joint line, or the medial or lateral tibial plateaus. No tenderness over the proximal fibular head. No tenderness, fullness, or mass of the popliteal fossa. No quadriceps tenderness. No laxity of the ACL, PCL, MCL, or LCL. May note no collateral ligament laxity to valgus or varus stress. Neg Lachman/Drawer signs. Neg McMurray. Neg Apley compression and/or distraction. Distal motor and neurovascular status intact

(cont.)

KNEE PAIN (cont.)

JOINT ASPIRATION PROCEDURE NOTE

Procedure explained and consent obtained. Pt was placed in a sitting/supine position with knee supported and slightly flexed. The skin was prepped with povidone–iodine solution and cleansed with NS. The site was anesthetized with 1% lidocaine ( ) mL with good anesthesia. The lateral/medial joint space was entered using an 18- or 20-gauge needle. A slight "give" was appreciated as the needle entered the joint capsule. ( ) mL fluid (clear, cloudy, bloody, fat globules) was aspirated. The needle was removed and a dry, sterile antibiotic dressing was placed over the puncture site and a compression dressing (e.g., Ace wrap) was applied. Joint fluid was sent for CBC with diff, glucose, protein, crystals, and C&S. Tolerated procedure well with no complications

X-RAY NOTE

For example, right knee series was done to R/O fracture or dislocation. There was no fracture, no effusion, dislocation, soft tissue swelling, or FB noted

SPLINT NOTE

There was no neurovascular compromise after splint/immobilizer application; the splint/immobilizer was in good alignment and the pt had good sensation and capillary refill at the time of discharge

KNEE X-RAY ORDERING CRITERIA

- Age 55 or older
- No TTP of knee other than patella
- PT of fibular head
- Inability to flex knee to 90°
- Inability to bear wt (four steps—unable to transfer weight twice onto each lower limb regardless of limping) both immediately and in ED

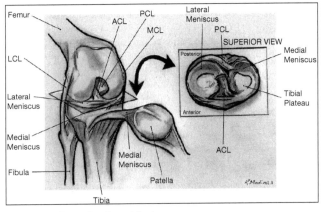

Anatomy and superior view of the knee

(cont.)

KNEE PAIN (cont.)

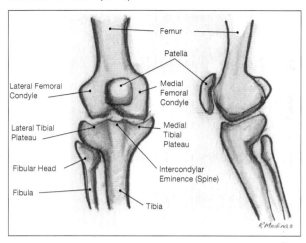

Frontal and lateral views of the knee

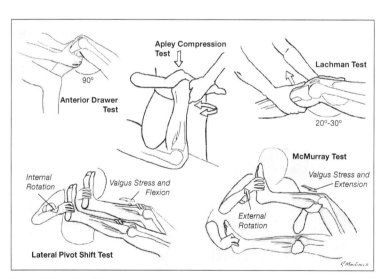

Provocative tests of the knee

(cont.)

KNEE PAIN (cont.)

DON'T MISS!

- Subtle FXs of tibial plateau, fibular head, small avulsion FX of proximal lateral tibia
- Widened joint space—unstable ligamentous injury
- If joint dislocation—delayed SXS of vascular injury
- Compartment syndrome
- Quadriceps rupture—be sure can extend and resist
- Look for other causes of knee pain (hip/back esp. peds)

● TIP

- If unable to bear weight—knee immobilizer, crutches, recheck 1 to 2 days. Exam deferred (McMurray and Apley man/tests) if pt in significant pain and is unable to perform test

DEEP VEIN THROMBOSIS

DVT RISK FACTORS

- Mild to severe leg pain and/or STS of calf, medial thigh, upper extremities
- Immobilization greater than 3 days, recent prolonged travel, hospitalization
- Surgery within past 4 weeks
- Recent plaster cast of lower extremity
- Active cancer
- Swelling of the entire leg, may be mild to severe: pitting edema in the affected leg. Calf swelling >3 cm when compared to unaffected leg. Superficial nonvaricose veins with palpable, tender cords

Adapted from Scarvelis, D., & Wells, P. S. (2006). Diagnosis and treatment of deep vein thrombosis. *Canadian Medical Association Journal, 175*(9), 1087–1092. doi:10.1503/cmaj.060366; Wells, P. S., Anderson, D. R., Rodger, M., Forgie, M., Kearon, C., Dreyer, J., . . . Kovacs, M. J. N. (2003). Evaluation of D-dimer in the diagnosis of suspected deep-vein thrombosis. *New England Journal of Medicine, 349*(13), 1227–1235. doi:10.1056/NEJMoa023153; Wells, P. S., Owen, C., Doucette, S., Fergusson, D., & Tran, H. (2006). Does this patent have deep vein thrombosis? *Journal of the American Medical Association 11, 295*(2), 199–207. doi:10.1001/jama.295.2.199

HX

- Older age: 60 years, obesity, smoking, sedentary/bed rest
- CVA, heart/resp failure, SLE, IBD, CA, DM, renal/hepatic failure
- Previous DVT/PE
- Recent surgery
- Trauma
- Cellulitis
- Use of hormones (e.g., estrogen therapy), hypercoagulopathy disorders

PE

- **General**: level of distress
- **VS and SaO$_2$**
- **Skin**: PWD
- **Extremities**: TTP calf or medial thigh—may be absent to severe; possible overlying warmth, erythema or discoloration or blanching of skin, gangrene, poor pulses, signs of compartment syndrome, Homan's sign (including pain with forced dorsiflexion of foot)

MDM/DDx

DVT caused by clot formation in the deep veins of an extremity can cause nonspecific pain and swelling or dislodge and travel to the lungs, leading to a life-threatening **pulmonary embolus**. Similar signs and symptoms can be caused **by super cial thrombophlebitis or varicose veins**. Soft tissue etiologies, such as local **hematoma** or **muscle injury**, should be considered. Erythema and swelling may also indicate **cellulitis**. Other systemic causes of edema include **hepatic** or **renal failure**. **Phlegmasia cerulea dolens** (painful blue inflammation) is a life-threatening condition that leads to extreme limb ischemia due to DVT. Consider in pts with severe leg pain and swelling, cyanosis, gangrene, compartment syndrome, and signs of shock. **Phlegmasia alba dolens,** or "milk leg," causes a whitish discoloration—if extensive, DVT leads to impaired arterial flow

(cont.)

DEEP VEIN THROMBOSIS (cont.)

MANAGEMENT

- Analgesia, ultz, anticoagulants, thrombolytics (see "Pulmonary Embolus")
- Smaller, isolated distal DVT may be treated with analgesia, ambulation, and weekly ultz.
- Complicated DVTs include HX of DVT or malignancy, >5 cm in length or 7 mm in diameter, multiple sites or near proximal veins

DICTATION/DOCUMENTATION

- **General**: alert and in acute distress
- **VS and SaO$_2$**
- **Skin: PWD, no cyanosis or pallor**
- **Extremities**: symmetry of R/L extremity when compared to the R/L. No STS or edema. No overlying erythema, warmth, discoloration. No lesions or break in skin integrity. Diameter of calves is _____ cm. Soft tissues of posterior lower leg are soft, supple, NT, and no palpable cords or evidence of thrombophlebitis. Medial thigh is without STS or TTP. Negative Homan's sign. Possible superficial thrombophlebitis with palpable, tender cords. No proximal lymphangitis or lymphadenopathy

◑ TIPS

- Be sure to check current renal status when considering the use of new anticoags (e.g., rivaroxaban or apixaban)
- Symptomatic patients with initial negative extremity ultrasound may require repeat imaging in 7 to 10 days

ANKLE/FOOT PAIN

HX

- Onset, duration, pain, F/C
- MOI—inversion "rolled," eversion, direct trauma, step from height, able to bear weight
- Associated injuries
- Previous injury/infection/surgery
- Recent quinolone use—tendon rupture or worsening myasthenia
- OA/RA
- HX gout/pseudogout

PE

- **General**: level of distress
- **VS and SaO$_2$** (if indicated)
- **Lower extremity—ankle**
- **Note**: compare with unaffected side; observe gait, ability to bear weight
- Obvious asymmetry, deformity/crepitus, STS/effusion, surface trauma, ecchymosis, open wounds, ulcers, erythema, warmth, dorsalis pedis/posterior tibial pulses; distal neurovascular status
- Extensive STS caused by crush injury—consider compartment syndrome STS, erythema, exudate, hypertrophy of nail or margins, subungual hematoma. Presence of tophi (gout).
- Distal neurovascular status
- TTP of talus, calcaneus, metatarsals 1 to 5, each MTP joint and IP joint, plantar/dorsal surface
- ROM: plantar/dorsiflexion, inversion/eversion
- ROM: flex/ext, inversion/eversion
- TTP or deformity over anterior ankle, med/lat malleolus, navicular, proximal fifth metatarsal, calcaneus, Achilles tendon, midfoot/toes TTP, STS, ecchymosis over deltoid ligament, TFL, PTFL, CFL
- Simmonds-Thompson test: absence of foot plantar flexion on calf compression is interpreted as positive test result, indicative of Achilles tendon rupture
- Squeeze test—pain along midshaft of fibula when compressed with tibia (high ankle sprain of syndesmosis)
- Talar tilt with valgus/varus stress
- Anterior drawer test
- Peroneal nerve: eversion/plantar flexion
- **Note knee pain**: STS, effusion, pain or deformity over proximal fibula (Maisonneuve FX: proximal fibular FX with medial malleolar injury)
- **Foot and toes:** check proximal fifth metatarsal
- **Examine knee and foot**: evaluate other knee, ankle, and foot/toes

(cont.)

ANKLE/FOOT PAIN (cont.)

ANKLE/FOOT X-RAY ORDERING CRITERIA

- Ankle x-ray: PT at posterior edge or tip of lateral malleolus, PT at posterior edge or tip of medial malleolus
- Inability to bear weight both immediately and in the ED
- Ordered if there is any pain in the midfoot zone and any of the following: PT at base of fifth metatarsal, PT at navicular. Inability to bear weight both immediately and in the ED.

Adapted from Stiell, I. G., Greenberg, G. H., McKnight, R. D., Nair, R. C., McDowell, I., Reardon, M., . . . Maloney, J. (1993). Decision rules for the use of radiography in acute ankle injuries. Refinement and prospective validation. *Journal of the American Medical Association, 269*(9), 1127–1132. doi:10.1001/jama.269.9.1127

MDM/DDx

Foot or ankle pain can affect any age group but older adults are more susceptible because of degenerative joint and soft-tissue disorders. MDM must consider both acute and chronic causes of pain. In addition to trauma, older adults must be evaluated for dermatological, vascular, or neurological etiologies for foot or ankle pain. Bony injuries include **FXs** or **dislocations**; most FXs of the toes and nondisplaced FXs of the metatarsals are not clinically significant. However, intra-articular, displaced, and multiple metatarsal FXs require prompt referral. Midfoot injuries should be evaluated for **Lisfranc sprain** or **fracture**. Injuries with neurovascular deficit, open **fractures, severe crush injury**, or concern for **compartment syndrome** are orthopedic emergencies. Overuse, direct, or indirect trauma to the foot can result in soft tissue injuries, such as **contusions, sprains, and tendonitis**, including plantar fasciitis or bone spurs. **Achilles tendon rupture** is more common in middle age but older people, especially men or those taking quinolones or steroids, are at increased risk. Soft tissue infections range from **ingrown toenails and cellulitis** to **diabetic ulcers**, a serious complication usually requiring hospitalization. Spontaneous pain, with swelling and erythema of first MTP joint, suggests **gout** (podagra). Other nonurgent causes of pain in the older adult include **hallux valgus (bunion)** or **hammertoe**. **Morton's neuroma** presents with a painful nodule on the ball of the foot, often between the third and fourth toes. Arterial flow is assessed by adequate capillary refill and dorsalis pedis and posterior tibial pulses. Diabetics and older adults with atherosclerosis are more prone to **arterial insufficiency** and **stasis dermatitis**. A symmetric loss of sensation and pain suggests **peripheral neuropathy; vasculitis** may cause asymmetric peripheral nerve pain or hypersensitivity. Ice, elevation, NSAIDs, and analgesia may help. Buddy tape toe FX, rigid ortho shoe, posterior mold, and crutches may also assist. Orthopedic consult for unstable or clinically significant FX. **Ingrown toenail:** warm soaks, NSAIDs, Abx, definitive toenail avulsion. **Diabetic ulcer infection:** saline dressing, possible debridement, control hyperglycemia, consider **cellulitis or** x-ray to R/O **osteomyelitis**. Vancomycin 20 mg/kg IV BID plus ampicillin/sulbactam 3 g IV or piperacillin/tazobactam 4.5 g IV QID. **Gout:** consider septic joint. NSAIDs, including indomethacin, analgesia, steroids, avoid alcohol and high-purine foods. Colchicine 1.2 mg PO, followed by 0.6 mg in 1 hour (review renal/hepatic function and recent meds for contraindications)

(cont.)

ANKLE/FOOT PAIN (cont.)

MANAGEMENT

- Trauma: ice, elevation, NSAIDs, analgesia. X-rays to R/O FX or dislocation. Air splint, brace, taping. Equine splint for Achilles tendon injury. Splint, crutches, NWB for severe sprain or FX. Gentle ROM, bear weight as tolerated. Orthopedic consult for unstable FX: disruption of mortise, FX/dislocation, bi- or trimalleolar FX
- Infection/Inflammation: (see "Knee Pain" for gout or joint infection) CBC with diff to evaluate leukocytosis or anemia; chemistries to detect hyperglycemia and renal function; wound culture; poss x-ray for FB, gas, osteomyelitis; wound debridement. Clindamycin or TMP/SMX (DS) if outpt; vancomycin **plus** Unasyn or Flagyl **plus** Cipro IV if admission. **Vascular**: arterial Doppler study for bilateral diminished pulses or delayed capillary refill. Ultz to R/O DVT for unilateral foot or ankle pain and swelling

DICTATION/DOCUMENTATION

- **General**: level of distress
- **VS and SaO$_2$**
- **Ankle/Foot**: pt is able to bear weight and ambulate without pain. The R/L ankle/foot is with/without obvious asymmetry or deformity when compared to the R/L ankle/foot. Pt can flex/ext, invert/evert. No obvious surface trauma, ecchymosis, or STS. No bony TTP over the medial or lateral malleolus. Anterior talofibular ligament, posterior talofibular ligament, calcaneofibular ligament NT, and without swelling. (May also be referred to generally as medial/deltoid or lateral ligaments.) NT or deformity of the midfoot or over the proximal fifth metatarsal. Good dorsalis pedis and posterior tibial pulses and sensation to light touch normal. Talar tilt test is negative for ligament laxity to valgus or varus stress. Negative anterior drawer. Peroneal nerve is intact with strong eversion and plantar flexion

X-RAY NOTE

There was no fracture, dislocation, soft tissue swelling, gas, or FB noted

SPLINT NOTE

There was no neurovascular compromise after splint application; the splint was in good alignment, and the pt had good sensation and capillary refill at the time of discharge

(cont.)

LOWER EXTREMITIES: Ankle/Foot Pain

ANKLE/FOOT PAIN (cont.)

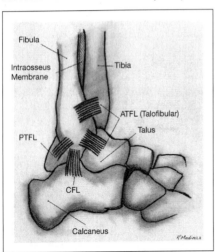

The anatomy of the ankle (lateral view)

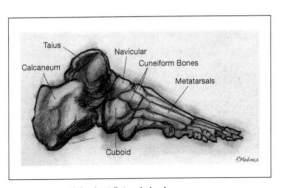

The anatomy of the foot (lateral view)

(cont.)

ANKLE/FOOT PAIN (cont.)

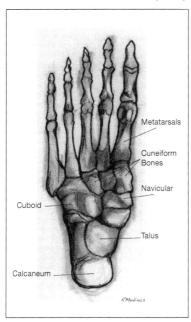

Metatarsals

Cuneiform Bones

Navicular

Cuboid

Talus

Calcaneum

R.Medina

Anatomy of the foot (superior view)

⊙TIP

- Include knee exam with attention to tenderness over proximal fibula. Include foot/ toes exam. If unable to bear weight—crutches, recheck 1 to 2 days. Look for associated injuries in older adults such as neck, lumbar spine, and pelvis

DON'T MISS!

- Peroneal nerve injury (occult injury)
- Achilles tendon rupture
- Check proximal fifth metatarsal or proximal fibular fracture

LACERATIONS/WOUNDS

HX

- Exact time of injury/delayed presentation/prior treatment
- MOI: blunt, penetrating, crush injury, organic matter, animal bite, FB
- Dominant hand, occupation
- Concern for elder abuse
- Puncture wound through tennis shoe (*Pseudomonas*)
- Contaminated with seawater
- Work-related history or exposure
- High-pressure paint gun, staple gun
- Closed-fist wounds
- Associated injury, self-inflicted wounds
- HX: comorbidities: DM, immunosuppressed
- Meds/Allergies/Immunizations (Td, Tdap)
- HX: diabetes, steroid use

PE

- **General**: level of distress, pain, F/C
- **VS and SaO$_2$**
- **Skin**: wound location, length, depth, linear, curvilinear, stellate, flap, jagged
    - Tissue loss, devitalized tissue, visible or palpable FB
    - Crush injury, exposed bone or tendon, active bleeding, STS, ecchymosis
    - Distal motor neurovascular status intact
    - Repeat motor exam under anesthesia and ROM
- **Note**: detailed motor neurovascular exam if injury to digit/extremity

MDM/DDx

Factors that may affect wound healing in older adults include general health status and nutrition. Wound healing may be impaired by arterial or venous insufficiency, neuropathy, inadequate perfusion, or underlying metabolic disease. Wounds are divided into types of repair: **simple, intermediate, or complex.** Anatomic location and wound length in cm must also be noted. Multiple wounds can be reported in total cm unless the wounds are of varying complexity. **Simple repair** includes closure of superficial wounds involving only the skin, regardless of length. Intermediate lacerations include approximation of skin and subcutaneous layer, galea, or superficial fascia. Simple wound closure that required extensive cleaning and removal of particulate matter may be classified as intermediate in some cases. **Complex repair** includes multiple-layer repair, debridement, extensive undermining, or placement of retention sutures.

MANAGEMENT

- Thorough wound irrigation and exploration with adequate hemostasis are the foundations of wound care. Identification of underlying deep structure injury or retained FB is essential for optimal wound healing. Wounds that may require specialty referral include:
    - Large avulsions or near amputations
    - Severe crush injuries and/or devitalized tissue involvement of eyelid tarsal plate or tear-duct system; auricular hematoma
    - Large cartilage defects
- X-ray for FB may be indicated. Update tetanus prophylaxis
- Consider Abx for contaminated wounds, delayed presentation, older adults, or immunosuppressed pts

(cont.)

LACERATIONS/WOUNDS (cont.)

SUTURE REMOVAL

- 4 to 5 days: eyelid, lip, face
- 4 to 6 days: pinna ear, neck
- 7 days: scalp/head
- 10 to 12 days: trunk or extremity
- 12 to 14 days: hand or foot. If wound is healing poorly or infected, consider retained FB

SUTURE SIZE

- 6.0 Face
- 5.0 Hand
- 4.0 Extremities

LACERATION PROCEDURE NOTE

Procedure explained and consent obtained. The wound was anesthetized with ( ) mL of good anesthesia. (Note local infiltration, field block, digital block.) Sterile drape and prep were done. Copious irrigation was done with NS and the wound explored. (Note whether able to visualize depth of wound.) There was no foreign body or deep structure injury noted. (Note whether examined under range of motion.) Wound edges were approximated with good alignment using (sutures, staples, skin adhesive, skin tapes). There were (number) of sutures/staples placed (type of suture). Type of dressing applied if done. Tolerated procedure well with no complications

DON'T MISS!

- Advise pt of possible retained FB—note in chart
- Open fracture, tendon injury, joint capsule disruption

(cont.)

LACERATIONS/WOUNDS (cont.)

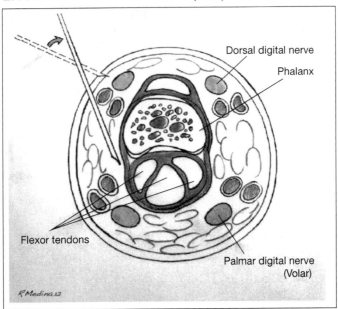

Cross-section of anatomy for digital nerve block

CUTANEOUS ABSCESS/CELLULITIS

HX
- Onset, duration
- F/C, N/V, nausea, vomiting
- Injury, insect, animal (e.g., dog, cat), human bite, FB, illicit drug use. History or exposure to complicated skin infections (MRSA), MRSA risk factors
- Current treatment
- Tetanus status
- Comorbidities: immunosuppressed (DM, Hep C, HIV), alcoholic, recent postop wound

PE
- **General:** F/C, malaise
- **VS and SaO$_2$**
- **Skin:** localized pain/tenderness, swelling, erythema, fluctuance, induration
- Pointing, drainage, palpable crepitus
- Central eschar formation
- Surrounding erythema, warmth
- Proximal lymphangitis, regional lymphadenopathy
- Distal edema
- Describe location, size, shape, consistency, margins
- Perform rectal exam if in perianal area—note fissures, tenderness, mass, fluctuance

MDM/DDx

As people age the skin is more fragile and peripheral circulation is often impaired, which increases the risk of soft tissue infections. Small abscesses without cellulitis usually require only simple I&D followed by supportive measures such as warm soaks. Midfacial infections are at risk for **cavernous sinus thrombosis. Extensive** or **multiple abscesses**, especially in immunocompromised pts, are clinically significant. **Perianal abscesses** are areas of concern because it is difficult to determine the extent of abscess formation and can lead to fistula formation. Other abscesses are caused by **hidradenitis suppurativa**, infected **sebaceous cysts, pilonidal cysts,** or **staph infections.** Consider infected lymph node versus abscess formation on the neck or groin areas. **Erysipelas** is a cellulitis that causes a painful, very red plaque with raised and sharply defined borders. Small areas of cellulitis without necrosis often improve with only a short course of oral antibiotics. Complex situations include large or **rapidly spreading cellulitis, failed outpt treatment, immunosuppression, or signs of sepsis**. Older pts are at risk for rapid deterioration from infection. Severe soft tissue infections may result in necrotizing fasciitis (rapidly spreading cellulitis with ulcers, necrosis, crepitus, bullae). Periorbital cellulitis (preseptal) must be evaluated for extension to orbital cellulitis. Erysipelas caused by group A beta-hemolytic streptococci is a painful infection that causes an area of erythema and swelling with a sharply demarcated border, usually on the legs or face

(cont.)

CUTANEOUS ABSCESS/CELLULITIS (cont.)

MANAGEMENT CUTANEOUS ABSCESS

- I&D is foundation of treatment
- Packing: none or wick only to keep wound open
- Warm soaks, NSAIDs
- Abx not usually indicated unless immunosuppressed, DM, MRSA, multiple abscesses, cellulitis. Consult for perirectal abscess

MANAGEMENT CELLULITIS

- Consider hyperglycemia
- Fever control, NSAIDs, analgesia, elevation, and warm soaks. Possible soft tissue x-ray or ultz to R/O FB or gas
- Abx (7–10 days): clindamycin 450 mg TID; doxycycline 100 mg PO BID; TMP/SMX (DS) 1 to 2 tabs PO BID; amoxicillin/clavulanate 875 mg PO BID; cephalexin 500 mg PO QID; dicloxacillin 500 mg PO QID; vancomycin 15 to 20 mg/kg IV QID; clindamycin 600 mg IV TID
- **Erysipelas**: penicillin 500 mg PO QID × 10 days or cephalexin 500 mg PO QID × 10 days or clindamycin 600 mg QID × 5 days then decrease to 300 mg QID
- Recheck 1 to 2 days, sooner if worse
- Admit for IV Abx if immunosuppressed, extensive, rapid spread, failed outpt, toxic

SUPERFICIAL CUTANEOUS ABSCESS I&D PROCEDURE NOTE

Procedure explained and consent obtained. The wound was anesthetized with ( ) mL good anesthesia. Sterile drape and prep were done. The fluctuant center was incised with #11 blade scalpel. A small/moderate/large amount of (exudate/blood/caseous material) was expressed or removed. The wound was probed for loculated areas and irrigated with normal saline. Note whether the wound was packed loosely with wick or left open. DSD was applied. Tolerated procedure well with no complications

DON'T MISS!

- Extensive or circumferential cellulitis with severe pain
- Necrotizing fasciitis—rapidly spreading erythema and pain within hours
- Orbital cellulitis
- Hand cellulitis

DECUBITUS

HX

- Age >70 years. Immobility, poor nutritional status. Altered mental status, use of restraints
- Impaired BMI
- Urinary and fecal incontinence
- PMH: CV, pulmonary, renal disease DM, CVA
- Fever and chills

PE

- VS and SaO_2
- Skin:
  - **Stage I:** pain in the area, but no open wounds or tears in the skin. Reddened skin that does not blanch. Skin temperature warm. Skin may feel firmer than the surrounding skin
  - **Stage II:** open skin, tender and painful. May look like an abrasion, blister, or an ulcer
  - **Stage III:** extension of the sore deeper in the tissue forming a crater. Fat may be visible
  - **Stage IV:** sore is deep and muscle, bones, joints, or tendons may be visible
- Describe location, stage, and size
- Perform rectal exam if in the perianal area

MDM/DDx

Pressure sores or decubitus ulcers are of concern because they can be a sign of poor nutrition or care. Stage III to IV can be sources of **infection and possible sepsis.**

MANAGEMENT

- Identify and document location. Stage the pressure sore. Record the size of the injured area. Estimate the depth
- Note any drainage if present. If bleeding is noted, obtain hemoglobin and hematocrit. Consider debridement of a small amount of tissue. If large amounts are present, consult surgery. Assess for cellulitis and treat if present. Referral for wound care if pt is discharged

DON'T MISS!

- Pressure sores as a source of sepsis
- Excessive blood loss from wounds that are bleeding; pressure sores as a sign of neglect

SEPSIS

Older adults can present with serious infections anywhere along a continuum and may progress from SIRS to sepsis and result in severe sepsis and septic shock

HX

- F/C, mental status changes
- Abd pain
- Indwelling urinary catheter, prosthetic device, heart valve replacement, long-term IV line
- Dementia, immobile, poor intake, dehydrated, malnourished, ETOH/drug abuse, polypharmacy
- Nursing home residence, recurrent hospitalization
- Recent UTI or kidney problems, GI tract disease, pneumonia
- Baseline functional status (outcome predictor)
- PMH: cancer, cardiac/renal/liver Dx, diabetes, obesity, alcoholism, endocrine deficiency, on steroids

PE

- **General:** toxic appearing, frail, AMS
- **VS and SaO$_2$:** fever <36°C or >38°C (97°F–100.40°F), heart rate (HR) >90, respiratory rate (RR) >20, SBP <90, pulse ox
- **Skin:** hot or cool skin, delayed cap refill, poor turgor
- **HEENT:**
  - **Head:** normocephalic
  - **Eyes:** pupils, PERRLA and EOMI, sunken
  - **Ears:** TMs and canals clear
  - **Nose:** patent
  - **Mouth/Throat:** dry lips and intraoral mucosa
- **Neck:** supple, no lymphadenopathy, no meningismus, no JVD
- **Chest:** CTA bilaterally or focal rales, tachypnea, accessory muscle use, decreased TV
- **Heart:** RRR, no murmurs, rubs, or gallops
- **Abd:** surface scars, soft/flat/distended; BS (absent ileus), guarding, rebound, rigid, tender, masses
- **Rectal:** exquisite tenderness (prostatic abscess), infected decubitus
- **GU:** perineal soft tissue infection, cellulitis, necrotic bullae (nec fasciitis), decreased urinary output
- **Back:** spinal or CVAT
- **Extremities:** moves all extremities, strength, sensation, distal pulses, mottling
- **Neuro:** alert, disoriented, obtunded, CN II–XII, focal neuro deficits

(cont.)

SEPSIS (cont.)

MDM/DDx

Rapid identification and immediate treatment of sepsis in the older adult is essential for survival. The clinical presentation is often vague and easily missed; sudden rapid deterioration and septic shock must be anticipated. Older adults are predisposed to sepsis because of immunosuppression, multiple comorbidities, cognitive or functional impairments, and repeated and lengthy hospitalizations. The mean age for severe sepsis is about 60 years, with the very old at great risk for death. Frequent sources of sepsis in older adults are **pneumonia** and **urosepsis**; nursing home residents are at an even greater risk. There are many other causes such as **meningitis** and **intra-abd abscess. Severe sepsis** involves organ dysfunction and can progress to **septic shock** with cardiovascular collapse. Consider conditions that mimic clinical presentation of sepsis such as **hemorrhage/hypovolemia, pancreatitis, PE, MI, DKA/HHS.** Mortality rate >50% in older adult pts who present in septic shock, which should prompt end-of-life considerations; consult with pt, family, social services, pastoral care

MANAGEMENT

- Protocol approach based on "International Surviving Sepsis" guidelines using preset bundles of diagnostic and therapeutic interventions. Sepsis management must start immediately upon pt presentation; triage time is "time zero" for initiation of treatment for early septic shock
- ABCs: initiate oxygenation and assisted ventilation as indicated; volume replacement (30 mL/kg crystalloid) guided by SBP as older pts may not have significant tachycardia; maintain preload to improve CO and watch closely for volume overload but continue fluids as hemodynamic status improves. Poss albumin 5% bolus
- Labs: FSBS, dip UA, CBC with diff, BMP, LFT/lipase, cardiac enzymes/trop, lactate, blood Cx ×2 before Abx, UA/Cx CXR (infiltrate, free air), EKG, poss CT brain/abd/pelvis
- Meds: identify source of infection and start Abx within 1 hour; broad spectrum. The empirical antimicrobial regimens should be based on pt factors, such as underlying comorbidities or immune-compromised states, site, and severity of infection; environmental factors, such as residence in nursing homes, history of repeated hospitalizations, and local factors like the expected microbiological organism and the antimicrobial susceptibility patterns. Vancomycin 1 to 2 g IV piggyback *and either* ceftriaxone 1 to 2 g IV or piperacillin–tazobactam 4.5 g IV. If concern for Gram neg infections, *add* gentamicin or ciprofloxacin/levofloxacin. Metronidazole plus either levofloxacin or ceftriaxone
- Vasopressors if no response to volume replacement. First choice is norepinephrine 0.05 mcg/kg/min IV. Epinephrine 0.05 mcg; kg/min; can *add* vasopressin 0.03 U/min to increase MAP. Possible dopamine, dobutamine as indicated. Consider IV steroids if no improvement with vasopressors
- CVP line placement and monitoring; arterial line if vasopressors needed
- Reassess: MAP goal 65 mmHg, CVP goal 8 to 12 mmHg, UOP >0.5 mL/kg/hr, improved lactate levels. Surgical consult if concern for intra-abd/pelvic infection. Remove any infected indwelling lines, and drain abscesses

⊙ TIPS

- Any altered mental status in the older pt requires an evaluation for a possible UTI or other source of infection such as pneumonia
- Older adults are less likely to have fever or chills when septic
- Bacteremia carries a high mortality in the older adult so there needs to be a high index of suspicion for it

(cont.)

SEPSIS (cont.)

DON'T MISS!

- Fahrenheit >38° or <36°; HR >90; R >20; B/P <90 new-onset AMS
- WBCs <4,000 or >12,000 or >10% bands; lactate >1 mmol/L

- Advanced directives or POLST/MOLST form, which can help direct the care of the critically ill older pt

HYPERTENSIVE URGENCY/EMERGENCY

HX

- Elevated B/P
- HA, blurred vision, confusion/ALOC, dizzy, fainting, seizure
- Chest pain/SOB
- Swelling or edema
- Muscle weakness, numbness, tingling, problems with balance or speech
- Changes in medication; medication withdrawal
- PMH: HTN, CVA, CVD
- Current B/P meds/compliance with meds
- Previous episodes of hypertensive crisis

PE

- **General:** alert, altered mental status, seizure
- **VS: B/P all extrems**
- **Skin:** PWD, rash
- **HEENT:**
    - **Head:** normocephalic, atraumatic
    - **Eyes:** PERRLA, sclera, conjunctiva, corneas, EOM, retinal changes papilledema, retinal hemorrhage/exudate
    - **Ears:** canals and TMs
    - **Nose:** drainage
    - **Face:** sinus tenderness, facial swelling, decreased pulsation or tenderness over temple
    - **Mouth/Throat:** MMM, condition of teeth
- **Neck:** supple, FROM, lymphadenopathy, meningismus
- **Chest:** CTA or rales, pulmonary edema (pink sputum if severe)
- **Abd:** soft, NT, back renal bruits
- **Extremities:** moves all extremities with good strength, distal motor/sensory intact, good pulses in all extremities
- **Neuro:** A&O ×4, GCS 15, CN II–XII, focal neuro deficit, DTRs, pathological reflexes, speech/gait, Romberg, pronator drift, speech clear, gait steady

MDM/DDx

Many people over 60 years have some degree of **systolic HTN** and almost all do by 75 years. In general, most pts with asymptomatic HTN do not require screening for acute target organ injury or treatment in the ED but should be referred for close follow-up by the primary care provider. Attempts to reduce long-standing HTN too quickly can precipitate ischemia. Appropriate management of elevated B/P depends on the ability to immediately differentiate hypertensive urgency from hypertensive emergency. **Hypertensive urgency** is HTN without end-organ damage and usually does not require initiation of treatment in the ED. A **hypertensive emergency** exists if there is evidence of end-organ dysfunction: brain, heart, kidneys. Evaluate for **hypertensive encephalopathy, CVA, intracerebral or subarachnoid hemorrhage, seizure, MI, acute left ventricular failure with pulmonary edema, aortic dissection, unstable angina pectoris, or acute renal failure**. Treatment is dependent on the presence or absence of target-organ involvement.

(cont.)

HYPERTENSIVE URGENCY/EMERGENCY (cont.)

MANAGEMENT

- **Asymptomatic HTN** with B/P >210 systolic or >120 diastolic: check chemistry for renal function; refer for outpt management. Consider initiating treatment if concern for poor outpt follow-up
- **Hypertensive urgency:** UA for hematuria, red cell casts or proteinuria, chemistries for renal function, EKG. Close follow-up 1 to 2 days
- **Hypertensive emergency:** ABCs, VS with appropriately sized B/P cuff, cardiac monitor. UA for hematuria, red cell casts, or proteinuria; chemistries for renal function, CBC for anemia, cardiac enzymes with troponin. EKG for evidence of acute MI, unstable angina, or left or right ventricular hypertrophy. CXR for pulmonary edema or cardiomyopathy. Noncontrast head CT scan for intracerebral hemorrhage or subarachnoid hemorrhage
- Medication goal: diastolic reduction to 100 to 110 mmHg within 2 to 6 hours; not more than 25% within minutes to 1 hour—even more caution with CVA. Rapid reduction required for aortic dissection; maintain adequate volume status
- Labetalol or nicardipine for encephalopathy, CVA, renal failure, or aortic dissection. Nitroprusside may be needed for dissection but avoid in renal failure; ACS: NTG, beta-blocker.

DICTATION/DOCUMENTATION

- **General:** awake and alert, not toxic appearing
- **VS:** no fever or tachycardia
- **SaO_2:** WNL
- **Skin:** PWD, no lesions or rash, no petechiae
- **HEENT:**
  - **Head:** scalp atraumatic, NT, no trigger points
  - **Eyes:** sclera and conjunctiva clear, corneas grossly clear, PERRLA, EOMI, no nystagmus, no ptosis, no photophobia, normal funduscopic exam, normal visual fields, IOP
  - **Ears:** canals and TMs normal
  - **Nose/Face:** no rhinorrhea, congestion; no frontal or maxillary sinus TTP; no asymmetry
  - **Mouth/Throat:** MMM, no erythema or exudate
- **Neck:** supple, FROM, NT, no lymphadenopathy, no meningismus
- **Chest:** CTA
- **Heart:** RRR, no murmurs, rubs, or gallops
- **Extremities:** moves all extremities with good strength, normal gait
- **Neuro:** A&O ×4; GCS 15, CN II–XII grossly intact. No focal neurological deficits. Normal muscle strength and tone. Normal DTRs, negative Babinski, normal finger-to-nose coordination or heel-to-shin glide. Speech clear, normal gait. Negative Romberg, no pronator drift

DIABETES: HYPERGLYCEMIC EMERGENCIES

HHS and DKA are serious diabetic emergencies that are associated with higher morbidity and mortality in the older adult. Both conditions are the result of a reduction in available circulating insulin and elevated levels of glucagon, cortisol, and catecholamines. The most significant factors for the development of either HHS or DKA are inadequate insulin therapy or underlying infection. HHS is more common in pts with type 2 DM while more pts with type 1 DM experience DKA.

Note: Consultation with a specialist and the use of evidence-based guidelines should be used as the science changes.

HX

- Onset: HHS develops gradually over days to weeks; DKA onset usually less than 24 hours
- Fever may be present if underlying infection; may be hypothermic as a result of vasodilation; severe hypothermia ominous. Increased thirst, urination, weight loss, weakness
- Neuro changes or coma more common in HHS: speech changes or muscle weakness, lethargy to coma, seizures, hemiparesis. Vomiting and diffuse abd pain frequent with DKA; hematemesis. Heartburn, abd bloating
- Recent illness or infection, poor oral hydration, immobility, dementia, surgery, comorbidities, drug use
- Meds that lower glucose tolerance or contribute to fluid loss: diuretics, niacin, glucocorticoids, antipsychotics, beta-blockers

PE

- **General:** alert, lethargic, confused, hallucinations, comatose, seizures, toxic appearing, signs of dehydration
- **VS and SaO$_2$:** fever or hypothermic, tachycardia, compensatory tachypnea, hypotension, hypoxemia
- **Skin:** PWD, cool/moist, hot, poor turgor, tenting, pallor, delayed cap refill, cyanosis, tenting of skin
- **HEENT:**
  - **Head:** atraumatic, NT
  - **Eyes:** sunken eyes, PERRLA, sclera, conjunctiva, corneas, EOM, fundi, nystagmus, visual field losses, eye deviation, hemianopsia
  - **Ears:** canals and TMs
  - **Nose:** drainage, congestion
  - **Face:** symmetry, normal strength and sensation
  - **Mouth/Throat:** MMM or dry cracked lips, possible acetone breath, dry or moist mucous membranes
- **Neck:** supple, FROM, lymphadenopathy, meningismus, JVD, or flat neck veins (dehydration)
- **Chest:** CTA, hyperventilation, tachypnea, Kussmaul respirations
- **Heart:** RRR, no murmur or gallop, tachycardia
- **Abd:** soft/flat/distended/diffuse tenderness BSA, guarding, rebound, rigid, pulsatile masses, scars, surface trauma, hernia
- **Back:** no spinal or CVAT
- **Extrems:** weak, thready pulses, muscle weakness, tetany
- **Neuro:** GCS 15, CN II–XII, focal neuro deficit, DTRs, pathological reflexes, speech/gait, myoclonic jerks, hemiparesis, seizures, decreased muscle tone

(cont.)

DIABETES: HYPERGLYCEMIC EMERGENCIES (cont.)

MANAGEMENT

- Management approach is similar for both HHS and DKA: aggressive volume replacement, correct hyperglycemia, and electrolytes
- Derangement, identify underlying infection
- **Volume**
  - IV NS bolus 1 L/hr initially; possible plasma volume expanders for hypovolemic shock
  - Estimated fluid volume deficit is often up to 10 L; replace 50% in the first 12 hours Consider central venous pressure monitoring to prevent fluid overload
  - Change to D5NS when blood sugar 250 to 300 mg/dL; monitor blood sugar level hourly
- **Insulin**
  - DKA: regular insulin 0.1 mg/kg IVP (if not hypokalemic) followed by continuous infusion of regular insulin 0.1 U/kg/hr
  - HHS: regular insulin infusion (0.1 U/kg/hr) only after volume replacement initiated and potassium >3.3 and urine output shows normal renal perfusion
  - If serum glucose does not fall by 50 mg/dL in first hour, insulin dose may need to be doubled every hour. When serum glucose 300 mg/dL, reduce insulin infusion to maintain serum glucose 250 to 300 mg/dL until mental status improves
- **Potassium**
  - Fluids, insulin, and correction of acidosis help correct elevated potassium level but need to manage resulting hypokalemia
  - Adequate renal function must be confirmed in HHS prior to potassium replacement therapy
  - Potassium level >5.0 mEq/L: monitor potassium level every 2 hours
  - Potassium level 3.3 to 5.0 mEq/L: 20 to 30 mEq potassium level in each 1 L NS to maintain potassium level between 4 and 5 mEq
  - Potassium level <3.3 mEq/L: 40 mEq potassium level until >3.3 mEq/L. Delay insulin infusion until potassium level + >3.3 mEq/L; watch for arrhythmia or cardiac arrest
- **Monitoring**
  - Chemistries every 2 to 4 hours until blood sugar is normal. Hypomagnesemia usually corrects with volume replacement; hypophosphatemia not routinely corrected unless tetany present. Monitor VS, cardiac rhythm, UOP frequently. ICU admission

(cont.)

DIABETES: HYPERGLYCEMIC EMERGENCIES (cont.)

DIAGNOSTICS

- Labs:
  - Blood sugar >600 mg/dL, absent to small serum ketones, serum pH >7.30, bicarbonate >15 mEq/L, serum osmolality >320 mOsm/kg
  - CBC: H&H elevated because of hypovolemia; elevated WBC because of infection, stress, dehydration BUN/creatinine: elevated. Ratio often over 30:1
  - Chemistries: blood sugar markedly elevated. Total body potassium is usually low regardless of presenting potassium level; risk of cardiac dysrhythmia with hypokalemia. Sodium may be elevated or decreased because of the osmotic effect of hyperglycemia, which draws water into the intravascular space. Hypomagnesemia is common. Elevated bicarbonate >15 mEq/L. Anion gap >12 mmol/L
  - Serum ketones: absent in HHS, present in DKA
  - ABGs: pH <7.30. VBG if normal SaO$_2$ on room air (0.03 pH units less than arterial)
  - UA: small ketonuria if dehydrated, specific gravity >1.035, pyuria, bacteria
  - Consider: serum lactate, blood/urine/sputum cultures, LFTs, lipase, cardiac enzymes and troponin, HbA1c as baseline; lumbar puncture if concern for CNS infection
- Imaging:
  - CXR to R/O infection
  - CT brain to R/O CNS cause of altered mental status
- Other diagnostic:
  - EKG: consider MI or PE as precipitating event for HHS; monitor peaked T waves with hyperkalemia; altered QT interval with calcium abnormalities

MDM/DDx

Acute **hyperglycemia** in older adults may be associated with either **HHS** or **DKA**. Immediate bedside blood sugar level should be obtained in any older pt who presents with altered mental status. **HHS** is a potentially life-threatening condition that presents with a dramatically elevated blood sugar level and has a mortality rate of 20% or higher in older pts. More prevalent in the disabled, demented, nursing home pts, obese, or those with comorbidities who have poor fluid intake and are easily dehydrated. Men and women are about equally affected but there is a disproportionate incidence among African Americans, Hispanics, and Native Americans. HHS is usually caused by poorly controlled blood sugar or undiagnosed **DM**; it is also often precipitated by illness or infection that causes dehydration or reduced insulin activity. **DKA** in older adults is usually caused by lack of insulin and classically presents with hyperglycemia (lower than HHS), ketonemia, and metabolic acidosis. DKA is also often precipitated by recent illness or stress such as infarction. Other causes of acidosis in older adults must be considered such as **starvation, chronic renal failure, salicylate, methanol** or **ethylene glycol ingestion** (antifreeze), and **alcoholic acidosis**. Many pts with DKA present with abd pain and must be evaluated for signs of **acute abd**. Decreased renal function in older pts leads to **hyperglycemia** and hyperosmolarity. The resulting osmotic diuresis and fluid shifts lead to **severe dehydration and metabolic derangement** resulting from fluid and electrolyte imbalance. The degree of hyperglycemia correlates well to the degree of dehydration. Renal failure, hypotension, coma, and hypothermia are poor outcome indicators. Other causes for altered mental status to consider include **pneumonia, UTI, pancreatitis, CNS dysfunction, DKA, intoxication, acute blood loss, CVA, and ACS**.

(cont.)

DIABETES: HYPERGLYCEMIC EMERGENCIES (cont.)

DICTATION/DOCUMENTATION

- **General:** level of distress, level of consciousness, improvement in baseline mental status
- **VS and SaO$_2$:** elevated temp or hypothermia, tachypnea, tachycardia, hypotension
- **Skin:** PWD. No diaphoresis, cyanosis, or pallor. Texture, turgor, tenting
- **HEENT:**
  - **Head:** normal, atraumatic
  - **Eyes:** not sunken, pupils PERRLA, EOMI, no nystagmus
  - **Ears:** TMs and canals clear
  - **Nose:** patent
  - **Mouth/Throat:** MMM or dry tongue, acetone odor of the breath reflecting metabolic acidosis
- **Neck:** supple, no lymphadenopathy, no meningismus, no JVD
- **Chest:** CTA bilaterally; tachypnea or hyperventilation (Kussmaul respirations)
- **Heart:** RRR, no murmurs, rubs, or gallops; tachycardia
- **Abd:** soft/flat/distended/diffuse tenderness, guarding, rebound, rigid, pulsatile masses, scars, surface trauma, hernia. BSA in all four quadrants
- **Back:** No CVAT
- **Extremities:** FROM, muscle tone and strength, reflexes
- **Neuro:** GCS 15, CN II–XII, focal neuro deficit, DTRs, Babinski, speech, myoclonus

❯ TIPS

- HHS
- Is more common in older pts with DM2 than DKA
- Increased because of poor PO fluid intake
- Anion gap formula: $(Na^+ + K^+) - (Cl^- + HCO_3^-)$

DON'T MISS!

- HHS as a cause of AMS or increase in confusion
- HHS can lead to sepsis (esp. from UTI)

HYPOTHYROIDISM

HX

- Complaints often very subtle, especially in the older adult
- Women >65 years
- Fatigue, loss of energy, lethargy/sleepy, withdrawn, depressed, emotionally labile, forgetful, impaired memory or concentration. Obtunded, seizure, comatose; possibly precedes psychosis. Decreased appetite, weight gain, constipation. Puffy face and hands, large tongue and swollen lips
- Dry skin, hair loss, muscle/joint pain, weak extremities, paresthesias, gait instability. Blurred vision, decreased hearing
- Feeling of fullness or pain in throat, hoarseness, painless thyroid enlargement. Cold intolerance, decreased perspiration
- PMH: thyroid disease, DM, autoimmune disease, use of radioactive iodine, hypothalamic-pituitary disease (central hypothyroidism), neck/chest irradiation
- Meds: noncompliance with thyroid meds. Beta-blockers, sedatives, narcotics, phenothiazines, amiodarone, interferon alfa, lithium, interleukin (IL)-2, rifampin, phenytoin, carbamazepine, phenobarbital
- FH: hypothyroidism

(cont.)

HYPOTHYROIDISM (cont.)

PE

- **General:** alert, disoriented, slowed speech and movements. Level of distress. Able to ambulate or ataxic. Appropriate hygiene
- **VS and SaO$_2$:** bradycardia. Decreased SBP, increased DBP. Hypothermia in severe cases
- **Skin/Hair:** PWD, rash, texture, and turgor. Coarse, brittle, straw-like hair; hair loss. Decreased perspiration, jaundice
- **HEENT:**
  - **Head:** normocephalic
  - **Eyes:** sclera and conjunctivae clear. PERRLA. EOMI, periorbital puffiness. Visual acuity if blurred vision
  - **Ears:** canals and TMs normal. Normal or decreased hearing
  - **Nose/Face:** rhinorrhea, dull facial expression, coarse facial features
  - **Mouth/Throat/Tongue:** MMM, tongue symmetrical, macroglossia. Teeth present or absent, posterior pharynx clear without erythema, lesions, exudate, or stridor, hoarseness, dysphagia, drooling
- **Neck:** supple, FROM. No meningismus or adenopathy, trachea midline. Carotids are equal. No bruits or JVD. Thyroid enlarged; simple or nodular goiter. Thyroidectomy scar
- **Chest:** normal AP diameter, no accessory muscle use. Good expansion without retractions. No tenderness. CTA, bilaterally with good tidal volume, or hypoventilation and respiratory depression and abnormal lung sounds
- **Heart:** RRR, no diminished or muffled heart tones (pericardial effusion), bradycardia. No murmurs, rubs, or gallops; peripheral pulses present and equal
- **Abd:** flat, soft, NT, or protruding. No masses, guarding, or rebound tenderness. BSA or hypoactive. No hepatosplenomegaly. No distension or ascites
- **Back:** no spinal or CVAT
- **Extremities:** FROM. Normal or decreased strength. No rigidity. No clubbing, cyanosis, or edema. Peripheral pulses intact, presence of vascular changes, varicose veins, vascular ulcers, pigmented skin, hair loss. Pitting or nonpitting edema in lower extremities. Sensation intact or decreased sensation
- **GU:** normal external genitalia without lesions or masses. No hernia noted. Note urinary/stool continence or incontinence
- **Neuro:** A&O ×4. GCS 15, CN II–XII grossly intact. Disoriented, slow to answer. No focal neuro deficits. Speech clear, gait stable or unable to ambulate. Muscle strength and sensation, able to move all extremities. Normal DTRs or hyporeflexia. No Babinski. Neg Romberg. Brief MME: year, date, month; location; three-word recall

(cont.)

HYPOTHYROIDISM (cont.)

MDM/DDx

Hypothyroidism is common in older adults and symptoms can be subtle. Many complaints are common in older adults such as fatigue, hearing loss, and dry skin. **Myxedema coma** is a rare metabolic and cardiovascular emergency caused by severe hypothyroidism that causes all body functions to slow. This crisis more often affects women and may be precipitated by underlying infection or stress and has a mortality rate of up to 80%. Pts often present with altered mental status, such as confusion or lethargy and sometimes coma. VS changes reveal hypothermia, bradycardia, hypotension, and respiratory depression. **Adrenal insufficiency** is a common comorbidity that must be considered. **Apathetic hypothyroidism** includes symptoms of depression, inactivity, withdrawn behavior, and lethargy; also associated with weight loss, constipation, muscle weakness, and cardiac symptoms. **Autoimmune thyroid disease (Hashimoto disease)** is the most common cause of hypothyroidism worldwide. In some pts with normal thyroid function, serious illnesses or sepsis can cause low total T4 levels without an increase in thyrotropin level. **Nodular thyroid disease** or **malignancy** should always be considered when nodules are palpated or a goiter is present

MANAGEMENT

- Myxedema coma
- ABCs with assisted/mechanical ventilation; venous access and careful fluid replacement; ICU admission. Warming measures: mortality rate related to degree of hypothermia. Correction of hyponatremia and hypoglycemia. Identify underlying infection or precipitating stressor
- **Labs:** CBC with diff, chem panel, LFTs, calcium, serum cortisol. TSH (thyroid stimulating hormone or thyrotropin), T3 (triiodothyronine), total and free T4 (thyroxine), TBG (thyroid-binding globulin), autoantibodies (anti-TPO, antimicrosomal, anti-Tg). Cultures for occult infection/LP. VBG/ABG. Toxicology
- EKG: bradycardia; low voltage if pericardial effusion
- CXR: cardiomegaly, pleural effusion, infiltrate
- Ultz: thyroid nodules
- Meds
  - Thyroid hormone replacement with either T3, T4, or both. Exact regimen varies and is controversial; follow hospital guidelines. Vasopressors (thyroid hormone replacement needed to be effective)
  - Hydrocortisone 100 mg IV q8h until adrenal insufficiency ruled out empiric Abx

(cont.)

HYPOTHYROIDISM (cont.)

DICTATION/DOCUMENTATION

- **General:** sleepy, lethargic, obtunded. Level of distress. Obese
- **VS and SaO$_2$:** hypothermia, bradycardia, tachycardia, low DBP
- **Skin:** PWD. Normal texture and turgor. No rash or lesions. No skin breakdown or decubitus ulcer, smooth skin. Or, coarse, dry skin, decreased turgor and moisture
- **HEENT:**
  - **Head:** normocephalic. Brittle, dry hair, hair loss
  - **Eyes:** sclera and conjunctivae clear. Corneal arcus senilis, cataracts. PERRLA EOMI. Diplopia
  - **Ears:** canals and TMs normal
  - **Nose/Face:** no rhinorrhea, face symmetrical
  - **Mouth/Throat:** MMM, tongue symmetrical. Teeth present or absent, posterior pharynx clear without erythema, lesions, or exudate
- **Neck:** supple without thyromegaly or adenopathy, trachea midline. No JVD. No noted dysphagia or drooling
- **Chest:** no accessory muscle use, normal AP diameter. CTA, no wheezes, rhonchi, rales. Normal TV
- **Heart:** RRR or bradycardia, no murmurs, gallops, or rubs; peripheral pulses present and equal. Normal S1 and S2
- **Abd:** protruding, soft, NT without masses, guarding, and rebound tenderness. BSA or hypoactive. No hepatosplenomegaly
- **Back:** no spinal or CVA tenderness
- **GU:** urinary/fecal continence or incontinence. Perineal skin breakdown. Ext: FROM, normal or decreased strength. Rigidity of limbs. No clubbing, cyanosis, or edema. Peripheral pulses intact. Vascular changes, varicose veins, vascular ulcers, pigmented skin, hair loss. Peripheral edema—pitting or nonpitting, anterior tibia or feet. Sensation intact or decreased
- **Neuro:** A&O ×4, GCS 15, CN II–XII grossly intact. No focal neuro deficits. Normal muscle strength and sensation. Speech clear. Gait steady or unsteady, assisted. Normal DTRs, negative Babinski. Normal finger-to-nose coordination or heel-to-shin glide. Negative Romberg, no pronator drift. Brief MME: year, date, month; location; three-word recall

▶ TIPS

- Consider hypothyroidism in older adults with new-onset arrhythmia, especially atrial fibrillation depression or decreased mental status, or failure to thrive
- Subtle complaints that are common in older adults may indicate hypothyroidism
- Watch for changes in T3 and T4 in hospitalized older adults with serious illness
- Recent hospitalization for an acute illness or use of glucocorticoid (e.g., epidural injection for pain management)
- Close outpt follow-up by PCP is essential if treatment for hypothyroidism begins in the acute setting

DON'T MISS!

- Altered mental status, hypothermia, bradycardia, hypotension, anemia, hyponatremia, hypoglycemia, depressed respiration (myxedema coma)
- Older adult pts with thyroidectomy scar, history of hypothyroidism, ^{131}I therapy

HYPERTHYROIDISM (THYROTOXICOSIS)

HX

- Signs may be very subtle in older adults. Age >60 years
- Nervous, anxious, irritable, agitated, hyperactive, tremors (may be diminished in older adults), trouble sleeping. Unexplained weight loss despite increased appetite
- Confusion, dementia, psychosis, seizure, coma; possible apathy and depression with toxic nodular goiter. Heat intolerance, sweating, thin skin, fine hair. Protruding eyes; dry, red, sensitive to light, blurred vision. Fatigue, muscle weakness
- Fever (may be very elevated), rapid, pounding heart beat; palpitations, SOB
- N/V; increasingly frequent stools; diarrhea, jaundice
- Swelling at the base of neck or palpable/visible thyroid gland; goiter
- Burning, itching, discolored and indurated skin of anterior tibia (pretibial myxedema). Also known as "orange peel/peau d'orange." Recent change in thyroid hormone replacement therapy; may result in toxic level HX or FH thyroid disease
- Smoker
- Emigration from countries with Hashimoto's disease prevalence
- Medications that contain iodine: amiodarone, interferon-alpha, multivitamins, cough syrup

PE

- **General:** level of distress, anxious, nervous, disoriented, hyperactive. Dressed appropriately or signs of poor hygiene
- **VS and SaO$_2$:** note vital signs and interpret as normal or abnormal, pulse ox interpretation, weight in kg (weight loss). Tachycardia or atrial arrhythmia. Systolic hypertension
- **Skin:** PWD, no rash. Good texture and turgor. Velvety, smooth skin, warm, moist skin. Jaundice. Pretibial myxedema
- **HEENT:**
  - **Head:** normocephalic
  - **Eyes:** sclera and conjunctivae clear. PERRLA. EOMI. Diplopia, proptosis, lid lag, stare. Check visual acuity if blurred vision
  - **Ears:** TMs and canals clear. Hearing normal
  - **Nose/Face:** no rhinorrhea
  - **Mouth/Throat:** MMM, tongue symmetrical. Teeth present or absent. Posterior pharynx clear without erythema, lesions, or exudate
- **Neck:** supple without meningismus or adenopathy, trachea midline. Carotids are equal. No bruits or jugular vein distention. No noted dysphagia or drooling
- **Chest:** normal AP diameter, no accessory muscle use. No tenderness. Lungs are clear, bilaterally with good tidal volume; or dyspnea, rales
- **Heart:** RRR or irregular and tachycardia. No murmurs, rubs, or gallops. Peripheral pulses present and equal
- **Abd:** flat, soft, NT or protruding without masses, guarding, rebound tenderness. BSA or hypoactive. No hepatosplenomegaly
- **Back:** no spinal or CVAT
- **GU:** normal external genitalia without lesions or masses. No hernia noted. Note urinary/stool continence or incontinence
- **Extremities:** limbs may look longer in proportion to the trunk. FROM, NT, strength and sensation, weakness, tremors, rigidity. No clubbing, cyanosis, or edema. Peripheral pulses intact (dorsalis pedal pulse may not be palpated, posterior tibial pulse present). Vascular changes, varicose veins, vascular ulcers, pigmented skin, hair loss
- **Neuro:** A&O ×4, GCS 15, CN II–XII, focal neuro deficit, DTRs, speech/gait. Romberg, pronator drift. Brief MME: year, date, or month; location; three-word recall

(cont.)

HYPERTHYROIDISM (THYROTOXICOSIS) (cont.)

MDM/DDx

Hyperthyroidism in the older adult is often very subtle and easily overlooked. Many complaints are common to a variety of other conditions or comorbidities. **Thyrotoxic crisis (thyroid storm)** is an extreme form of thyrotoxicosis with a very high mortality rate. This life-threatening condition requires a high index of suspicion and is diagnosed based on clinical findings because lab results are not readily available. This emergent problem is often precipitated by a stress, such as surgery, trauma, or serious infection in pts with untreated or partially treated thyrotoxicosis. Signs include hyperpyrexia >104, tachycardia, heart failure, N/V, agitatation, psychosis, seizures, and coma. **Graves' disease (diffuse toxic goiter)** is an autoimmune disorder that causes excessive thyroid hormone production. It is characterized by goiter, exophthalmos, and pretibial myxedema. **Toxic adenoma** and **multinodular goiter** are caused by hyperplasia of thyroid follicular cells; increased incidence with aging. **Apathetic thyrotoxicosis** may be seen in older adults with weight loss, apathy, and atrial fibrillation. **Thyroid malignancy** in the older adult should also always be considered. The antiarrhythmic medication amiodarone contains iodine and can cause **thyroiditis** in older adults even with normal thyroid glands. Some older adults have a **nodule** that produces excessive T3, which then suppresses thyroid gland function. Beware that the resulting low T4 level can be mistaken for hypothyroidism Graves' disease: low TSH, elevated T3 and T4, markedly elevated anti-TPO, +TSI; +RAIU; ultz increased flow. Thyroiditis: low TSH, elevated T3 and T4, −TSI; −RAIU; ultz decreased flow. Thyroid nodule: low TSH, elevated T3 and T4, −TSI; +/−RAIU

(cont.)

HYPERTHYROIDISM (THYROTOXICOSIS) (cont.)

MANAGEMENT

- Labs:
    - ABCs, venous access and fluid replacement (caution in CHF), D5NS for glucose replacement, cooling measures; identify underlying infection or precipitating stressor; ICU admission
    - CBC with diff, chem panel, LFTs, calcium, cortisol level, cultures. TSH (thyroid stimulating hormone), free T3 (triiodothyronine) and T4 (thyroxine), TSI (thyroid-stimulating immunoglobulin), anti-TPO (anti-thyroid peroxidase) test
    - Most specific autoantibody test for autoimmune thyroiditis: ELISA for anti-TPO antibody. RAIU test
- EKG: tachycardia, AFib CXR: infiltrate, CHF
- Imaging: ultz, CT, thyroid scan, RAIU
- Meds:
    - Beta-blocker to control adrenergic excess such as tachycardia or arrhythmia; caution if CHF present. Propranolol 1.0 mg IV over 10 minutes or 60 to 80 mg PO/NGT q4 to 6h; consider atenolol, esmolol, or diltiazem based on specific pt medical history
    - Thionamide to block new hormone synthesis. Propylthiouracil (PTU) 600 to 1,000 mg then 200 mg PO/NGT/PR q4 to 6h. PTU will also block T4 to T3 conversion
    - Methimazole 20 mg PO/NGT/PR q4 to 6h for severe but not life-threatening cases. Longer acting than PTU
    - Glucocorticoids to reduce T4 conversion to T3. Dexamethasone 1 to 2 mg IV q8h or hydrocortisone 300 mg IV bolus followed by 100 mg q8h
    - Iodine blocks new hormone synthesis and hormone release—wait at least 1 hour after thionamide. SSKI 5 gtts PO q6h or Lugol's solution 10 gtts PO TID. Avoid potassium iodine if on amiodarone. Consider lithium in pt allergic to iodine
    - Acetaminophen for hyperpyrexia. Avoid ASA
    - Diuretics if indicated
    - Abx as indicated
- Surgical thyroidectomy: large goiters, severe ophthalmopathy, refuse RAI, refractory amiodarone-induced hyperthyroidism. Urgent operative intervention may also be indicated for rapid correction of unstable cardiac condition caused by hyperthyroidism

(cont.)

HYPERTHYROIDISM (THYROTOXICOSIS) (cont.)

DICTATION/DOCUMENTATION

- **General:** level of distress, anxious, nervous, hyperactive, hygiene
- **VS and SaO$_2$:** tachycardia, irregular, HTN
- **Skin:** PWD. Normal texture and turgor. No rash or lesions. No skin breakdown or decubitus ulcer. Smooth, velvety, moist skin. No jaundice
- **HEENT:**
  - **Head:** normocephalic
  - **Eyes:** sclera and conjunctivae clear. Corneal arcus senilis, cataracts. PERRLA EOMI. Diplopia, proptosis, ptosis, stare
  - **Ears:** canals and TMs normal
  - **Nose/Face:** no rhinorrhea, face symmetrical
  - **Mouth/Throat:** MMM, tongue symmetrical
  - Teeth present or absent, posterior pharynx clear without erythema, lesions, or exudate
- **Neck:** supple without thyromegaly or adenopathy, trachea midline. No bruits or jugular vein distention. No noted dysphagia or drooling
- **Chest:** no accessory muscle use, normal AP diameter. CTA, no wheezes, rhonchi, rales. Normal TV
- **Heart:** RRR or tachycardia, irregularity, no murmurs, gallops, or rubs; peripheral pulses present and equal. Normal S1 and S2
- **Abd:** protruding, soft, NT without masses, guarding, and rebound tenderness. BSA or hypoactive. No hepatosplenomegaly
- **Back:** no spinal or CVA tenderness; GU: urinary/fecal continence or incontinence. Perineal skin breakdown
- **Extremities:** FROM, normal or decreased strength. Rigidity of limbs. No clubbing, cyanosis, or edema. Peripheral pulses intact. Vascular changes, varicose veins, vascular ulcers, pigmented skin, hair loss. Peripheral edema, pitting or nonpitting, anterior tibia or feet. Sensation intact or decreased
- **Neuro:** A&O ×4, GCS 15, CN II–XII grossly intact. No focal neuro deficits. Normal muscle strength and sensation. Speech clear. Gait steady, unsteady, assisted. Normal DTRs, negative Babinski. Normal finger-to-nose coordination or heel-to-shin glide. Negative Romberg, no pronator drift. Brief MME: year, date, month; location; three-word recall. If indicated, that is, "What is the year, date, or month? Where are you—hospital or department?" Cranial nerves II to XII intact. Motor and sensory intact

(cont.)

HYPERTHYROIDISM (THYROTOXICOSIS) (cont.)

○ TIPS

- Identification of thyrotoxic crisis made based on clinical findings and high index of suspicion
- Vague nonlocalizing symptoms or any change in usually stable older adults should prompt concern for thyroid dysfunction
- Recent hospitalization and/or treatment for acute illness can trigger acute hyperthyroidism
- Amiodarone can cause thyroiditis in older adults
- A plan for transition of care must be implemented for older adults tested or treated for hyperthyroidism in the acute setting to be followed up by primary care

DON'T MISS!

- Classic triad: hyperpyrexia, tachycardia, altered mental status ranging from agitation to coma
- Amiodarone as a cause of changes in thyrotropin
- New-onset AFib or heart failure may be caused by hyperthyroidism

HYPONATREMIA/HYPERNATREMIA

TYPES OF HYPONATREMIA

- **Hypotonic:** inadequate salt intake. Excessive losses (sweating, GI loss) replaced with hypotonic fluids. Renal salt loss (adrenal or pituitary insufficiency, renal disease)
- **Hypertonic:** impaired water and sodium excretion (CHF, renal or liver failure)
- **Euvolemic:** increased total body water compared with normal total body sodium. Inappropriate release of ADH sodium level so no volume depletion (pulmonary infection, malignancies, meds)

CAUSES OF HYPONATREMIA BASED ON VOLUME STATUS

- **Hypovolemia:** most common; both sodium and water low; fluid loss from V/D, dehydration, malnutrition
- **Hypervolemia:** both sodium and water high; CHF, cirrhosis, renal failure
- **Normovolemia:** both sodium and water normal; water intoxication, SIADH, thyroid Dx

HX

- Wide range of SXS
- HA, N/V/D, weak, fatigue, irritability, restless, malaise, muscle spasm, cramps
- Recent fever, illness, poor volume intake
- Altered mental status, lethargy, seizures, coma
- Dementia, long-term care facility resident, immobility, restricted access to water
- Recent surgery or hospitalization—infusion of hypotonic fluids
- Tube feedings: high glucose and protein
- Malnutrition
- Psychiatric: compulsive water intake
- ETOH—specifically beer (free water rich and solute poor)
- Meds: OTCs, antipsychotics/SSRIs/sedatives, diuretics, NSAIDs, salt tablets
- Extreme exercise
- HX sodium imbalance, CHF, renal or hepatic failure, pneumonia, neurologic disorders, TBI, SAH, tumors, pituitary disorders, DI (lithium, dopamine, or rifampin use, contrast agents), seizures
- Dietary HX: salt, protein, water intake

(cont.)

HYPONATREMIA/HYPERNATREMIA (cont.)

PE

- **General:** alert and oriented, oriented/disoriented/ALOS. May be delirious and/or combative
- **VS:** note vital signs and interpret as normal or abnormal, pulse ox interpretation, weight in kg. Orthostatic vital signs
- **Skin:** warm, dry, pink without rash. Good texture and turgor or poor, tenting
- **HEENT:**
  - **Head:** normocephalic
  - **Eyes: sunken eyes.** Sclera and conjunctivae clear. PERRLA. EOMI
  - **Ears:** patent canals. Tympanic membranes clear
  - **Nose/Face:** without rhinorrhea
  - **Mouth/Throat:** mucous membranes moist or dry. Tongue symmetrical. Teeth present or absent. Posterior pharynx clear without erythema, lesions, or exudate
- **Neck:** supple without meningismus, thyromegaly, or adenopathy, trachea midline. Carotids are equal. No bruits or jugular vein distention. No noted dysphagia or drooling
- **Chest:** normal AP diameter and no accessory muscle use noted. Good expansion without retractions. No tenderness. CTA, bilaterally with good tidal volume. Moist rales
- **Heart:** RRR, no murmurs, rubs, or gallops; peripheral pulses present and equal. An S_4 may be heard in healthy older people, which is suggestive of decreased ventricular compliance and impaired ventricular filling
- **Abd:** flat, soft, NT or *protruding* without masses, guarding, and rebound tenderness. BSA or hypoactive in all four quadrants. No hepatosplenomegaly
- **Back:** without spinal or CVA tenderness
- **Musculoskeletal:** limbs look longer in proportion to the trunk. Decreased tensile strength may be noted, caused by age or chronic disease such as osteoarthritis
- **GU:** normal external genitalia without lesions or masses. No hernia noted. Urinary continence or incontinence
- **Rectal:** normal tone or incontinent of stool. No rectal wall tenderness. Stool is brown and heme negative
- **Extremities:** FROM. Good to decreased strength bilaterally. Evidence of upper and lower extremity rigidity. No clubbing, cyanosis, or edema. Peripheral pulses intact, dorsalis pedal pulse may not be palpated, posterior tibial pulse present. Presence of vascular changes, varicose veins, vascular ulcers, pigmented skin, hair loss. Sensation intact
- **Neuro:** pt is alert, oriented or disoriented, dressed appropriately or signs of poor hygiene, such as lack of bathing, dirty hair and nails, clothes not clean; engaging, in no acute distress. Speech clear. Brief MME if indicated, that is, "What is the year, date or month? Where are you—hospital or department?" Three-word recall. Cranial nerve II to XII intact. Motor sensory exam nonfocal. Moves all extremities. **Gait:** steady, unsteady. **Romberg:** normal or abnormal

(cont.)

HYPONATREMIA/HYPERNATREMIA (cont.)

MDM/DDx

Sodium is essential to maintain normal osmotic pressure and acid/base balance; the concentration of sodium in the blood is a balance of water and sodium. Older adults are particularly susceptible to hyponatremia because of impaired water metabolism, decreased sensation of thirst, declining renal function, and responsiveness to ADH. Hospitalized older pts, especially those in long-term care facilities, are at increased risk for water and sodium imbalances. A normal sodium level is 135 to 145 mEq/L. **Hyponatremia <135 mEq/L** is usually associated with decreased osmolality <275; a problem with water retention rather than too little salt. Severe hyponatremia is a serum sodium concentration less than 120 mEq/L. Excessive fluid loss resulting from **vomiting** or **diarrhea** is a common cause. **Inadequate renal function, CHF,** and **cirrhosis** or hormonal imbalances caused by **adrenal insufficiency** or **hypothyroidism** can cause hyponatremia. Also, movement of sodium into interstitial spaces (third space) resulting from conditions such as **pancreatitis, peritonitis,** or severe **burns.** Very low sodium levels should prompt concern for **SIADH,** a pathological elevation of ADH and hyponatremia. Consider SIADH in older adults with dementia, tumors that secrete ADH, brain infections or subarachnoid hemorrhage, lung infections like TB or taking thiazide diuretics, ACE inhibitors, anticonvulsants, or SSRIs. **Iatrogenic hyponatremia** is a concern in older adults receiving hypotonic IV fluids; accidental or psychiatric **water intoxication** can also occur. Other conditions cause a false low sodium, such as **hyperglycemia,** which corrects as the glucose level normalizes. Overt neurologic symptoms caused by very low serum sodium levels (<115 mEq/L), which can result in intracerebral osmotic fluid shifts and brain edema. Hyponatremia can cause sudden death from seizures and lead to severe neurological impairment. **Hypernatremia >145 mEq/L** in older adults is caused by limited access to fluids and is more likely in those with cognitive impairment, immobility, or in long-term care living. Symptoms are evident with a rapid rise in sodium >158 mEq/L. Causes include any reason for loss of thirst, GI losses caused by severe diarrhea or laxative use, osmotic diuresis caused by severe hyperglycemia (DKA or HHS), diabetes insipidus, or occasional infusion of hypertonic solutions. Insensible fluid loss and sweating caused by hyperthermia contributes to hypernatremia. Medications can increase sodium levels (e.g., lithium, colchicine, rifampin, gentamicin). Loop diuretics, such as thiazides, can lead to fluid losses. Rapid recognition of the cause of hypernatremia can prevent morbidity and mortality. When serum sodium abnormality is identified, it is important to differentiate underlying causes based on osmolality to direct treatment. There are risks involved in the correction of sodium imbalance and abnormal lab levels should first be verified

(cont.)

HYPONATREMIA/HYPERNATREMIA (cont.)

MANAGEMENT

- After ABCs, initial treatment measures vary significantly and are based on type of sodium imbalance and directed toward the underlying cause of fluid and electrolyte imbalance
- Fluids: IV 0.9% NS if signs of hypovolemia, check orthostatic VS. Use hypertonic saline (0.3%) for severe neuro changes or seizures—calculate and use very carefully in older adults. Fluid restriction, loop diuretics (furosemide) for volume overload. Monitor I&O. Asymptomatic pts with hyponatremia, restrict oral intake to <1 L/d)
- Labs:
  - CBC with diff, chemistries
  - Serum osmolality: normal osmolality with low sodium (280–295 mOsm/kg): elevated protein or lipids. Low osmolality (<280 mOsm/kg): excessive fluid intake, renal/liver/thyroid Dx, SIADH, CHF. Elevated osmolality (295 mOsm/kg): osmotic load of hyperglycemia or mannitol administration
  - Urinary osmolality >100 mOsm/kg means impaired kidney ability to excrete free water; also initiate 24 hours of urine collection
- **Cautious hyponatremia correction** if indicated: 0.5 mEq/L increases every hour to start, do not increase by more than 10 mEq/L in 24 hours. Potassium replacement and correction of hyperglycemia if indicated
- **Hypernatremia and hyperglycemia with DM**, caution when using a glucose-containing replacement fluid but the appropriate use of insulin will help during correction
- The safety and effectiveness of AVP receptor agonists and Declomycin in older adults with hyponatremia is not known; consult before using EKG, CXR, noncontrast CT brain
- Possible dialysis for hypernatremia with pulmonary edema and heart failure
- Consultation and admission for close monitoring

(cont.)

MISCELLANEOUS: Hyponatremia/Hypernatremia

HYPONATREMIA/HYPERNATREMIA (cont.)

DICTATION/DOCUMENTATION

- General: alert and oriented, well appearing, appropriately dressed, oriented in no acute distress. No ALOS, irritability, lethargy, confusion, seizures, cognitive impairment. Dressed appropriately, or poor hygiene. Level of distress
- VS and SaO$_2$
- Skin: PWD, no lesions or rash. Good texture and turgor. No skin breakdown or decubitus ulcer
- HEENT:
  - Head: normocephalic, atraumatic
  - Eyes: sclera and conjunctivae clear. PERRLA. EOMI
  - Ears: patent canals. Tympanic membranes clear
  - Nose/Face: without rhinorrhea, face symmetrical
  - Mouth/Throat: mucous membranes are moist. Tongue symmetrical. Teeth present or absent, upper or lower plates, with or without significant decay. Posterior pharynx clear without erythema, lesions or exudate
- Neck: supple without any thyromegaly or adenopathy, trachea midline. No bruits or jugular vein distention. No noted dysphagia or drooling
- Chest: CTA, no accessory muscle use, normal AP diameter
- Heart: RRR, no murmurs, rubs, or gallops, peripheral pulses present and equal
- Abd: +BSA, protruding, soft, NT without masses, guarding and rebound tenderness. No HSM
- GU: urinary continence or incontinence. Perineal skin breakdown
- Rectal: no rectal wall tenderness. Stool is brown and heme negative
- Back: no spinal or CVAT
- Extremities: moves all extremities well with good strength, distal motor/sensory intact, and symmetrical, good pulses. No cyanosis, clubbing, edema, venous stasis
- Neuro: A&O ×4, GCS 15. CN II–XII intact. Speech clear. Brief MME if indicated, that is, "What is the year, date, or month? Where are you—hospital or department?" Three-word recall. Motor sensory exam nonfocal. Moves all extremities. Gait: steady, unsteady. Balance: normal or abnormal

▶ TIPS

- Older adults, especially with cognitive impairment, have a decreased thirst sensation
- Review baseline sodium: many older adults function well with baseline hyponatremia (128–130)
- Review meds: antidepressants can cause hyponatremia, carefully consider discontinuing or whether tapering is needed
- Consider consultation for end-of-life care or palliative care consult for pts with end-stage renal, cardiac disease, and/or malignancies

DON'T MISS!

- Pts with cognitive impairment taking psychotropic medications "off-label" to manage their behaviors
- Pts in long-term care facilities with an inc risk of developing hypernatremia because of immobility, cognitive impairment, and less access to fluids
- Impaired ability of the aging kidney to concentrate urine can result in free water loss and hypernatremia
- What sodium level is NORMAL for the pt? Important to review previous labs if available since this abnormal may be normal for the pt

MALTREATMENT

HX

- Limited resources to provide care for the pt
- Decreased functional ability of the pt
- Disability, frailty, cognitive impairment
- Caregiver stress, family stressors such as job loss
- Family conflict, history of family violence or abuse
- Isolation of the pt or caregiver or both
- Dependency of the caregiver on the pt
- Misuse of pt's assets
- Reports of abuse and neglect by the pt or others
- Pt left alone for long periods of time
- Lack of food or controlled environment for living
- Repeated ED visits; repeated hospital admissions
- Evidence of misuse of pt's assets
- Self-neglect—pt lives in isolation and chooses to endure and accept maltreatment

ASSESSMENT QUESTIONS TO CONSIDER

- How safe is the current environment that the older pt must return to? Should the pt be removed until there has been an assessment?
- Are there services available to provide support and care for an older adult?
- What is the status of the older adult's caregivers? What is the caregivers' physical and mental status?
- Does the situation require an immediate referral to adult protective services, home health assistance, crisis management, or admission to the hospital?

(cont.)

MALTREATMENT (cont.)

PE

- **General:** alert, disoriented, confused, tremulous, arousable, agitated, lethargic, stuporous, delirious, comatose. Recognition/interaction with family members or significant others. Hygiene, including hair and nails, inappropriate dress; appearance of clothing, trauma; odors (ETOH, acetone, almonds), signs of malnutrition
- **VS and SaO$_2$:** fever/hypothermia, brady/tachycardia, resp depression, hypo/hyperventilation
- **Skin:** texture, turgor—signs of dehydration, malnutrition, rash, petechiae/purpura, jaundice, bruise and bruise patterns, pressure ulcers, burns, signs of restraint on upper and/or lower extremities
- **HEENT:**
    - **Head:** surface trauma
    - **Eyes:** PERRLA, fixed/dilated, icterus, EOMI, ptosis, fundi (papilledema, retinal hemorrhage), periorbital edema
    - **Ears:** canals patent, hemotympanum, CSF leak
    - **Nose:** CSF leak
    - **Face:** symmetric, weakness
    - **Mouth/Throat:** gag reflex, tongue symmetry
- **Neck:** meningismus, nuchal rigidity, thyroid
- **Chest:** CTA
- **Heart:** RRR, resp effort
- **Abd:** soft, NT, pulsatile mass, ascites, hepatomegaly, suprapubic TTP or distension, fecal impactions
- **Extremities:** FROM, NT, strength and sensation, weakness, tremors, asterixis (liver hand flap), rigidity, contractures, fractures, or fractures in various stages of healing
- **Rectal:** tone, occult blood, melena
- **Neuro:** A&O ×4, GCS 15, CN II–XII, focal neuro deficit, DTRs, pathological reflexes, speech/gait, Romberg, pronator drift, speech clear, gait steady, spontaneous or uncontrolled movements, abnormal posturing, flaccid

MDM/DDx

MDM includes ruling out trauma, such as head or cervical spine injury; evaluate for hip and/or pelvic fractures, evaluate for fractures in various stages of healing, multiple bruises without cause, and bilateral bruises on the upper torso, as well as unexplained falls. Presence of disease that may be causing altered mental status (see "Delirium and Dementia"). Assess for signs of infection, such as UTI or pneumonia. Assess ability for pt to participate in activities of daily living, current social situation, and support systems.

(cont.)

MALTREATMENT (cont.)

MANAGEMENT

- Identification of significant injuries
- CT head/neck
- X-rays: CXR, hip/pelvis
- EKG
- CBC, chem panel, UA/Utox
- Measurable medication levels (as indicated)
- ABGs 9 (as indicated)
- Psychological or crisis assessment
- Report maltreatment as dictated by the state in which one practices
- Consults as needed
- Refer to home health

DICTATION/DOCUMENTATION

- **General:** alert and oriented, confused, unresponsive. No odors. VSS, no fever or tachycardia. **Presence of family or significant others and pt's and family's response. Describe any signs of maltreatment**
- VS and SaO$_2$
- **Skin:** PWD, no lesions or rash, no surface trauma noted. **Location of bruises, evidence of physical restraint, especially around wrists and ankles**
- **HEENT:**
    - **Head:** scalp atraumatic, NT
    - **Eyes:** sclera and conjunctiva clear, corneas grossly clear, PERRLA, EOMI, no nystagmus or disconjugate gaze, no ptosis. Corneal reflex intact. Fundoscopic exam
    - **Ears:** canals and TMs normal. No hemotympanum or Battle's sign
    - **Nose/Face:** atraumatic, NT, no asymmetry
    - **Mouth/Throat:** MMM, posterior pharynx clear, normal gag reflex, no intraoral trauma
- **Neck:** supple, FROM, NT, no lymphadenopathy, no meningismus
- **Chest:** CTA, no wheezes, rhonchi, rales. Normal TV, no retractions or accessory muscle use. No respiratory depression
- **Heart:** RRR, no murmurs, rubs, or gallops
- **Abd:** soft, NT, pulsatile mass, ascites, hepatosplenomegaly, suprapubic TTP or distension, pelvis stable or unstable
- **Back:** without spinal or CVA tenderness
- **Extremities:** moves all extremities with good strength, distal motor neurovascular intact. Area of injury—see specific injury descriptions
- **Neuro:** A&O ×4, GCS 15, CN II–XII grossly intact. No focal neurological deficits. Normal muscle strength and tone. Normal DTRs, negative Babinski, normal finger-to-nose coordination or heel-to-shin glide. Speech, gait, Romberg neg, no pronator drift.

⊙ TIP

- Be aware of individual state requirements for reporting suspected or confirmed maltreatment

END-OF-LIFE CARE

HX

- Out/in hospital resuscitation of cardiopulmonary arrest
- Injuries incompatible with life
- CHF, COPD, cancer, renal failure, CVA
- Dementia, delirium, anxiety
- Frailty, fatigue, weakness
- Pain
- N/V, D/C
- Dyspnea
- Advanced directives in place
- Physical or medical orders for life sustaining treatments (MOLST or POLST forms)

PE

- **General:** ALOC, difficulty finding words, short sentences, delayed or inappropriate responses, verbally unresponsive, signs of pain, such as grimacing or tension in forehead, between eyebrows
- **VS and SaO$_2$:** fever/hypothermia, brady/tachycardia, resp depression, hypo/hyperventilation, hypotension
- **Skin:** pale, diaphoretic, mottling, peripheral cyanosis
- **HEENT:**
  - **Eyes:** PERRLA, fixed/dilated, icterus, EOMI, ptosis, fundi (papilledema, retinal hemorrhage), periorbital edema, loss of ability to close eyes, whites of the eyes showing
  - **Nose:** CSF leak
  - **Face:** symmetric, weakness
  - **Mouth/Throat:** loss of ability to swallow, secretions, gurgling
- **Chest:** change in ventilatory rate—increasing first, then decreasing, abnormal breathing patterns, periods of apnea, Cheyne–Stokes respirations, agonal breathing
- **Abd:** soft, NT, pulsatile mass, ascites, hepatomegaly, suprapubic TTP or distension, fecal impactions
- **Extremities:** weakness, tremors, flaccidity, nonpalpable peripheral pulses
- **Rectal:** incontinence of bowel or bladder
- **Neuro:** decreasing level of consciousness, agitation, restlessness, purposeless movement, repetitive movements, moaning and groaning, unresponsive

MDM/DDx

Actively dying: signs of actively dying such as **altered mental status, respiratory dysfunction, dysphagia, coughing, choking, loss of gag reflex, altered respiratory pattern, apnea, loss of bowel and bladder control, signs of pain.** Need for **palliative care for symptom management:** shortness of breath, pain, anxiety, nausea and vomiting, constipation, and fatigue

(cont.)

END-OF-LIFE CARE (cont.)

MANAGEMENT

- Treatment based on symptoms identified
- Consult: palliative care team
- Disposition: admit to hospital, home health referral made to which agency
- Hospice evaluation
- Determine whether actively dying: identify pt and family wishes, evaluate POLST or MOLST forms; consult palliative care team or hospice if available
- Symptom control for a pt who is actively dying
- Terminal secretions: glycopyrrolate subQ or IV 0.1 mg; atropine sulfate subQ IV 0.1 mg or sublingual 1 gtt (1% ophth solution)
- Agitation: lorazepam or midazolam
- Pain management: morphine sulfate; hydromorphone
- Prepare the family and allow the family to be present with support
- Identify religious or cultural practices of the pt and family. Allow and accommodate as much as possible

Symptom Management For The Nonactive Dying Patient

Symptom	Management
Pain	Consider nonpharmacologic pain management methods such as ice, heat, positioning For opioids use algorithms that are available for both acute and chronic pain Use an equianalgesic dosing table Calculate initial dose of an opioid based on whether the pt is opioid naïve or tolerant Consider the effects of advanced age, as well as renal and hepatic impairment, when selecting a medication Evaluate the need for onset of pain relief and choose the appropriate route of administration and the pharmacokinetics of the drug-peak effect of the medication Consider the side effects of the medications chosen, that is, nausea, vomiting, respiratory depression, constipation Consider nonopioid medications, such as gabapentin and NSAIDs, when appropriate
Nausea and Vomiting	Identify the cause when possible, though at times in this pt population, it is not always clear; causes may include bowel obstruction, anxiety, chemo-therapeutic agents, increased ICP from metastasis Medications that are used are based on what the cause of the symptom is but include: anxiolytics, octreotide, hydration, steroids, antihistamines, and anticholinergics
Constipation	Identify the cause—bowel obstruction, medication side effects—especially opioids Management can include increased fluid intake, increase in physical activity, medications such as stimulant laxatives, osmotic laxatives, and lubricant stimulants

(cont.)

END-OF-LIFE CARE (cont.)

Symptom	Management
Diarrhea	Identify cause—medication side effects; infection, chemotherapy related changes in the GI tract Management can include—rehydration; evaluation and management or electrolyte imbalance; medications such as loperamide, diphenoxylate/atropine, and tincture of opium; severe secretory diarrhea may be treated with octreotide
Fatigue and Weakness	Look for causes: side effects of medications, disease treatments. Treatment should include both pharmacological as well as nonpharmacological methods. Examples of pharmacological approaches include dexamethasone and methylphenidate. Nonpharmacological includes physical and occupational therapy, hydration, and review of medications to adjust medications that can be causing fatigue and weakness when possible
Anxiety	Identify any participating factors that may have caused the pt or family to seek treatment in the ED Situational factors, such as fear of diagnosis and the treatment that may be needed, impending life changes, death Symptom-related factors including pain, nausea, dyspnea; treatment may include benzodiazepines, but should be used only on a limited basis Relaxation techniques and referral for long-term interventions are better for the pt and family
Dyspnea	Causes—disease process—bronchospasm, hypoxia, pleural effusions, pulmonary edema or embolus, thick secretions, anemia, myocardial infarction psychosocial—anxiety, fear Treatment—identification of the shortness of breath, oxygen, opioids—especially oral morphine—anxiolytics. Nonpharmacological methods—sensation of cool moving air—fan, positioning the pt, unobstructed view of window or door, noninvasive ventilation
Delirium	Delirium is defined as a transient, usually reversible, cause of cerebral dysfunction, and manifests clinically with a wide range of neuropsychiatric abnormalities. It can occur at any age, but it occurs more commonly in pts who are older and have compromised mental status

Source: Adapted from Bryant, E. (2013). Rapid palliative care assessment. In P. Sandre & T. Quest (Eds.), *Palliative aspects of emergency care* (pp. 17–22). Oxford, UK: Oxford University Press.

(cont.)

END-OF-LIFE CARE (cont.)

DICTATION/DOCUMENTATION

- **General:** alert and oriented, confused, unresponsive. No odors. VSS, no fever or tachycardia. Description of the pt related to the presenting symptom, that is, actively vomiting, pacing, grimacing, agitated. Pain assessment level
- **VS and SaO$_2$**
- **Skin:** PWD, no lesions or rash, no surface trauma noted
- **HEENT:**
    - **Head:** atraumatic, NT
    - **Eyes:** sclera and conjunctiva clear, corneas grossly clear, PERRLA, EOMI, no nystagmus or disconjugate gaze, no ptosis. Corneal reflex intact. Fundoscopic exam
    - **Ears:** canals and TMs normal
    - **Nose/Face:** atraumatic, NT, no asymmetry
    - **Mouth/Throat:** MMM, posterior pharynx clear, normal gag reflex, no intraoral trauma
- **Neck:** supple, FROM, NT, no lymphadenopathy, no meningismus
- **Chest:** CTA, no wheezes, rhonchi, rales. Normal TV, no retractions or accessory muscle use. No respiratory depression
- **Heart:** RRR, no murmurs, rubs, or gallops
- **Abd:** soft, NT, pulsatile mass, ascites, hepatosplenomegaly, suprapubic TTP or distension, pelvis stable or unstable
- **Back:** without spinal or CVA tenderness
- **Extremities:** moves all extremities with good strength, distal motor neurovascular intact. Area of injury—see specific injury descriptions
- **Neuro:** A&O ×4, GCS 15, CN II–XII. Focal neurologic deficits. Muscle strength and tone. DTRs, Babinski reflex

❯ TIPS

- ABCD
    - **Assessment**, which provides immediate assessment of palliative care needs of unstable pts/advance care plan in place?
    - Better symptom management while in the ED
    - Caregivers—who can make the decision and is there documentation available?
    - Decision-making capacity—can the pt make his or her own decisions?

Source: Adapted from Bryant, E. (2013). Rapid palliative care assessment. In P. Sandre & T. Quest (Eds.), *Palliative aspects of emergency care* (pp. 17–22). Oxford, UK: Oxford University Press.

Take care when administering opioids to avoid opioid toxicity. This results from accumulation of the metabolites. Signs of toxicity include tremors, myoclonic jerks, or seizures. Rotating the opioids that are used may decrease these symptoms; if there is not enough time,, then a benzodiazepine may be used to alleviate symptoms

(cont.)

END-OF-LIFE CARE (cont.)

WITHDRAWAL OF CARE IN THE ED

Before Any Withdrawal of Care (e.g., Extubation) Prepare Family
1. Identify the family's and pt's wishes.
2. Review any advanced directives or POLST/MOLST forms to establish DNR status.
3. Explain to the family what is going to be done.
4. Allow the family to see the pt. Encourage them to talk and touch the pt.
5. Be sure that the family understands that many times even when treatment is stopped, that is, ventilators turned off, endotracheal tubes removed, vasopressor medications stopped, the pt may not die immediately.

Prepare the ED Team Who Has Been Working With the Pt/Family
1. Discuss the plan of care.
2. Review how symptoms will be managed.

Steps to Withdraw
1. Turn off alarms, remove pt from cardiac monitor.
2. Ensure that the family is safe, that is, seated if needed.
3. Allow all family members who want to be present. Ask about and allow any religious representatives or cultural practices to be provided.
4. Encourage the family or others to talk and touch the pt.
5. Maintain an IV for symptom management.
6. Manage symptoms before extubation, that is, excessive secretions, gasping respirations.
7. Decrease oxygen to 21%.
8. Deflate ETT cuff and turn off the ventilator.
9. Gently clear any secretions.
10. Clinician should remain close by to support family, assess and manage any symptoms.
11. After death has occurred allow the family to take the time needed with the pt.
12. Offer information about what will happen next—medical examiner may need to be contacted, notification of funeral home, bereavement care.

Sources: Adapted from Bryant, E. (2013). Rapid palliative care assessment. In P. Sandre & T. Quest (Eds.), *Palliative aspects of emergency care* (pp. 89–98). Oxford, UK: Oxford University Press; *Geriatric review syllabus: A core curriculum in geriatric medicine.* New York, NY: American Geriatrics Society.

DISPOSITION/TRANSITION OF CARE

The care of older adults in the ED/urgent care setting is a significant challenge to healthcare providers, including the conclusion and transition of their care. It is especially important that care of older adult pts be safely transferred from the ED back to the primary care provider. The primary care provider needs to know what tests have been ordered, the results, and especially any change in medications

KEY ELEMENTS

- Admission and discharge planning
- Discharge diagnosis
- Medication reconciliation
- Medications administered in the ED including
  - Indications for the medication
  - Dosage (total amount given)
  - How administered
  - Adverse reactions
- Education provided to the pt and family about the medication
  - Need for monitoring of the medication
  - Scheduling of any monitoring, that is, PT/INR
- Tests performed
  - Copies
  - Computer access
- Referral tracking
  - Specialists
  - Home health agencies
  - Hospice care
- Assessment of functional status and cognitive function in pts over the age of 65
- End-of-life care discussions
- Completion of advanced directive forms
  - MOLST (Medical Orders for Life Sustaining Treatment)
  - POLST (Physician Orders for Life Sustaining Treatment)
  - These forms outline pt's or both pt's and family's wishes at the end of life. The forms address "attempt to resuscitate" or DNR; comfort care, limited interventions; or all interventions; use of antibiotics; use of a feeding tube; and use of intravenous fluids.
- Was the PCP contacted or an attempt to communicate with PCP made during the ED visit?
- Verbal hand-off to care facility

DICTATION/DOCUMENTATION

- Should reflect the key elements of the admission or discharge plan, including medication reconciliation, medication administration while in the ED, cognitive and functional assessments for a pt over 65 years of age, diagnostic tests performed and results, referral to any specialists, disposition location if different from where the pt presented from, and any follow-up that might be needed or arranged
- A discharge form should be produced with key elements addressed for the pt, family, and PCP
- PCP contacted or an attempt was made
- Follow-up care

(cont.)

DISPOSITION/TRANSITION OF CARE (cont.)

Sample Documentation—Older Adult Disposition/Transition of Care

Key Element	Selected Item
Diagnosis	Fall Altered mental status UTI
Cognitive Assessment	Cognitive function (Cognition)

	LEVEL OF CONSCIOUSNESS
	    Alert, drowsy, obtunded, comatose
	ORIENTATION
	    Person, time, place, situation
	ATTENTION
	    May be obvious
	    If not obvious:
	    Repeat six digits forward, four in reverse
	    Arithmetic: two digits
	    Serial 7s from 100
	    Count backward from 100
	MEMORY
	    Immediate
	    Three words or objects at 1 and 5 minutes
	    Recent
	    Events of the last few hours or days R/O confabulation by asking again
	    Remote
	    Past medical history
	(FUND OF) INFORMATION
	    Should be appropriate to pt's age, education, social situation
	    Famous people
	    Current events
	    Local geography

Functional Assessment Comments should be made about the pt's functional ability. Several scales have scoring systems (e.g., Barthel Index of ADLs)	Multiple scales available but some basic elements include: • Toileting • Feeding • Dressing • Grooming • Physical ambulation • Bathing • Instrumental ADLs Ability to use the phone Shopping Food preparation Housekeeping Laundry Mode of transportation Responsibility for own medications Ability to handle finances

(cont.)

DISPOSITION/TRANSITION OF CARE (cont.)

Key Element	Selected Item
Medication Continuity	Statement about how medications were reconciled while in the ED Statement about any changes made in pt's medications, including the added or deleted medications, the pt's or family's understanding about the medication changes
Test Continuity	Statement about test ordered/statement of test results Statement about with whom the results were discussed Statement plan of care for follow-up for abnormal results
Consultation Continuity	Statement about who the pt was referred to and why Any information that would include whether the specialist has been contacted by the ED and what information was given to the pt and/or family about the need for a referral or consultation
Prognosis and Goals of Care	Statement about plan of care
Planned Interventions	Referral to home health or hospice Durable medical equipment (e.g., oxygen started) Wound care
Advanced Directives	Code status discussion Completion of MOLST or POLST forms Consultation with palliative or hospice care
Discharge and Disposition Plan	Home with caregiver Return to care center (SNF or assisted living) Mode of transportation Contact made with primary care provider and plan discussed caregiver issues

Source: Adapted from Terrell, K. M., & Miller, D. K. (2006). Challenges in transitional care between Nursing Homes and emergency departments. *Journal of the American Medical Directors Association*, 7(8), 499–505.

○ TIPS

- Communication with primary care can improve the implementation of post-ED visit care plans and assist in preventing any unnecessary ED visits
- Medication reconciliation at the time of discharge (e.g., new meds) can prevent med errors and increase med compliance. Timeliness of availability and ED record transmission can greatly improve the transition of care, preventing ED readmissions

INDEX